Launching and Leading Change Initiatives in Health Care Organizations

Launching and Leading Change Initiatives in Health Care Organizations

Managing Successful Projects

DAVID A. SHORE

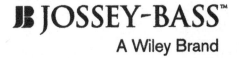
JB JOSSEY-BASS™
A Wiley Brand

Published by Jossey-Bass
A Wiley Brand
One Montgomery Street, Suite 1200, San Francisco, CA 94104-4594—www.josseybass.com

Jossey-Bass books and products are available through most bookstores. To contact Jossey-Bass directly call our Customer Care Department within the U.S. at 800-956-7739, outside the U.S. at 317-572-3986, or fax 317-572-4002.

Wiley publishes in a variety of print and electronic formats and by print-on-demand. Some material included with standard print versions of this book may not be included in e-books or in print-on-demand. If this book refers to media such as a CD or DVD that is not included in the version you purchased, you may download this material at http://booksupport.wiley.com. For more information about Wiley products, visit www.wiley.com.

Library of Congress Cataloging-in-Publication Data
Shore, David A., author.
Launching and leading change initiatives in health care organizations: managing successful projects / David A. Shore.—First edition.
    p.; cm.
  Includes bibliographical references and index.
  ISBN 978-1-118-09914-8 (cloth)—ISBN 978-1-118-41892-5 (pdf)—
ISBN 978-1-118-41598-6 (epub)
  I. Title.
  [DNLM: 1. Health Services Administration. 2. Organizational Innovation. 3. Planning Techniques. 4. Program Development. W 84.1]
  RA971
  362.1068—dc23

2013047962

Printed in the United States of America

FIRST EDITION

HB Printing   SKY10073091_041624

CONTENTS

LIST OF FIGURES AND TABLES

Figures

Tables

To my parents, Ruth and Milton Shore,
who embody every positive quality described in this book

PREFACE

ANY ORGANIZATION primarily does two things. It conducts its regular business. It also changes that business from time to time. In other words, its activities consist of operations and innovation. Leaders must always strike a balance between the two. Nevertheless, when an organization's environment is changing rapidly, it must innovate a lot. That is the situation health care organizations find themselves in today. If you are in health care, as the saying goes, you are seeing change.

How do organizations innovate? They launch initiatives. Change events. Projects. The vocabulary differs from one organization to another. Health care professionals will have no difficulty knowing what I am talking about, whatever the terminology. Something is changing pretty much all the time. Whatever it is, there's a team working on it.

As part of my work—beginning at the Harvard School of Public Health and continuing in other contexts—I developed a program on launching and managing projects. My colleagues and I have taught this program in numerous health care systems and in countries around the world. I have also taught seminars to professional associations, to conference groups, and in other settings. Every time we conduct the program, I make a point of asking the attendees to list some of the initiatives and projects they are involved in, and the list always astonishes me. One participant was trying to speed up turnaround time at his hospital's lab. Another was hoping to improve linen-loss management. A third was involved in creating a new Pain Management Center. Another was working on replacing the organization's financial system. The initiatives are big, small, and every size in between. They are long term and short term. They are in various stages of completion. Most of all, they are numerous.

When I ask participants how many projects they themselves are involved in, the answers typically range from six to twelve.

It is not surprising that projects have proliferated so widely in health care, given that the sector is evolving so quickly. New technologies appear regularly. Cost pressures are intensifying. All of health care's many stakeholders—patients, clinicians, administrators, payers, regulators, and so on—want to see improvements. The recent reform law in the United States, the Patient Protection and Affordable Care Act, popularly known as Obamacare, has already begun to affect health care organizations. For example, the act calls for more accountable care organizations (ACOs) and provides incentives for their creation. As a result, hospital systems, physician practices, and insurance networks all around the country are launching projects to turn themselves into ACOs. Like any change initiative, the movement toward ACOs can be thought of as an uncertain, risk-bearing experiment. Organizations have options in regard to their participation in the ACO program, however, with the "classic" option offering less risk and less potential reward, and the "premier" option offering more of both. This trade-off between risk and reward applies to many projects, not just ACOs.

It is essential for every stakeholder that well-conceived projects accomplish their objectives. Any change initiative's goal, after all, is to improve things, and health care badly needs improvement. Unfortunately, the failure rate of health care projects is high. Some projects crash and burn. Others peter out and are abandoned. Still others linger on indefinitely, never quite achieving their goals but never quite dying, either. I will offer some statistics about failure rates later in the book, but for the moment consult your own experience. Of all the projects you have been involved in, how many failed? How many are in trouble right now? Few of the leaders I speak with in the sector can answer "none" to either question.

Projects fail, of course, for many reasons. But my research and experience suggest one underlying malady that has infected nearly every dead or dying project: a poor launch. Whatever the specifics of an ailing project's diagnosis, the trouble was almost always built in from the beginning.

In noting the importance of a project's inception, I find that I have considerable support among the world's great thinkers. "Success depends upon previous preparation," said Confucius; "Without such preparation there is sure to be failure." Plato put it only slightly differently: "The beginning is the most important part of the work." An African proverb says, "If you want to know the end, look to the beginning." It has even been noted that Barack Obama, in implementing health care reform, would do well to heed the advice of the only other U.S. president to hail from the state of Illinois. "Give me six hours to chop down a tree," said Abraham Lincoln, "and I will spend the first four sharpening the axe."

Stephen R. Covey, the best-selling author of such books as *The 7 Habits of Highly Effective People*, elaborated on Lincoln's notion with a homely anecdote. A man walks to work and sees another man sawing a tree. On his way home from work, the same man is still sawing the same tree. The first man asks, "Have you thought of sharpening your saw?" The sawyer replies, "I don't have time to sharpen my saw. I am too busy sawing this tree."[1]

Where change initiatives are concerned, sharpening the saw—or the axe—is the difference that makes the difference.

To be sure, there are plenty of people in the business world who would discount the importance of spending so much time getting ready. "Ready, fire, aim" has become a mantra for many action-oriented managers—or, as Nike says, "Just Do It."[2] That may work in an Internet-based business such as Facebook, where product engineers can put something up on the website to see if it has the desired effect, and then make a change if it doesn't. But the approach doesn't work in health care. Too much is at stake. Errors are too costly, in lives as well as in resources. Besides, the evidence for the importance of good first-mile preparation is overwhelming. If I were to add an aphorism of my own, it might be this: "Initiatives don't end poorly—they begin poorly." Or maybe this: "With projects, the end depends on the beginning." Certainly the importance of a good launch resonates with the people in health care organizations who are actually involved in projects. One group of program participants, who happened to be in Illinois, presented me with a framed copy of Lincoln's quote about sharpening the axe. That, they said, was the single most important idea they took away from our several days together.

WHO SHOULD READ THIS BOOK

Anyone who leads or manages a health care initiative will benefit from this book. The book will also greatly benefit those who serve on project implementation teams. I say that with some assurance because so many of my students, executive education program participants, and clients have told me that they find the ideas and methodologies helpful. These students and professionals come from diverse roles in health care. They are physicians, nurses, and therapists. They are managers and administrators. Many are senior executives.

The people in this last group, senior leaders, have a special responsibility for starting projects right. If they don't provide the necessary support, it will be hard for even the best-intentioned project manager to achieve the hoped-for results. This is a lesson any of us could learn from W. Edwards Deming, the famous apostle of manufacturing quality, who died in 1993 at the age of ninety-three.

In the mid-1980s, Toyota was making serious dents in the market share of Detroit's Big Three—General Motors, Ford, and Chrysler. The Japanese company's chief advantage lay in its exceptional manufacturing quality. Toyotas didn't break down as often as other cars. They lasted longer. Their fit and finish, to use the auto industry's term, was far better. Deming had tried to interest U.S. automakers in his ideas about quality decades earlier, but had received a chilly reception. He ended up spending much of his working life in Japan, teaching quality principles to Toyota and other Japanese manufacturers.

Donald Petersen, who was chief executive of Ford from 1985 to 1989, watched an NBC special on Deming one night. As the story goes, he called his head of quality (who had never heard of Deming) and said, "We have to get this guy in here." Deming agreed to come on one condition: that Ford's top thirty leaders participate in his first seminar.[3]

With all the leaders gathered, Deming began his presentation. About halfway through, Petersen's secretary came in and handed him a note. Petersen left the meeting. Deming promptly took a chair and sat down. People in the audience assumed he must be tired—after all, he was already an elderly man. But fatigue wasn't the issue. Deming said to the group, "If Mr. Petersen has something more important than quality to attend to, don't you think we should wait for him?" After that, nobody left the room. Senior leaders in health care would do well to translate this lesson to the context of change management in health care.

Health care projects depend on astute management of change. But more than anything else, they depend on leaders who pay attention, who understand the importance of starting right, and who know how to launch projects that succeed. That is why I am hopeful that senior leaders of every sort of health care organization will read this book and take its lessons to heart. If leaders can increase the percentage of successful projects, patients and practitioners everywhere will be better off. So will the organizations that depend on these projects for innovation. As will the leaders themselves, for they will be accomplishing their goals rather than running down perpetual blind alleys.

Part 1 of this book lays the groundwork for my method. It looks at health care through the lens of change initiatives and thus managing change. It examines the fundamentals of these initiatives and outlines the criteria for success and failure. It explores what an organization must put in place if its projects are to get off the ground during that essential first mile.

Part 2 focuses on selecting the right projects, which is one of the two most important tasks of the first mile. Most health care organizations have scores of projects under way at the same time. It's a sort of "spray-and-pray" approach: if we try enough initiatives, maybe some will work out. I argue for a far more systematic method of selecting and supporting projects. It is not that I expect every one to succeed; the world is too uncertain for that. But I do want every project to be scrutinized, and then supported if it passes scrutiny. The chapters in this part offer a set of tools with which organizations can assess, approve, and set priorities for their portfolio of projects—and then review the projects as they proceed to see how well they are doing.

Part 3 dives into the other essential task of the first mile: choosing the right people. At many organizations, the same twenty or thirty or forty people always seem to wind up on project teams. They are the people leaders think of in connection with change. They are the ones who say, "Yes, sure, I can do that," rather than "Sorry, I'm too busy." The result is that this group of well-meaning, overworked individuals can't possibly devote the time required by all of their projects. Most already have a full-time "day job" anyway. Again, I advocate a more systematic approach in which organizations help people gain the skills necessary for projects, keep a database of individuals and the initiatives they are working on, and build effective teams of people with complementary skills.

Throughout, the book distills the mistakes of many organizations' initiatives so that you do not have to repeat them. The common theme is simplicity itself: ensuring that your projects start right so that they will end right. I hope you find it useful.

David A. Shore
Boston, Massachusetts
February 2014

NOTES

1. Stephen R. Covey, *The 7 Habits of Highly Effective People: Powerful Lessons for Personal Change* (1990; repr., New York: Free Press, 2004).
2. Robert Goldman and Stephen Papson, "Suddenly the Swoosh Is Everywhere." In *Nike Culture: The Sign of the Swoosh* (London: Sage, 1998), 19–20.
3. Andrea Gabor, *The Capitalist Philosophers: The Geniuses of Modern Business—Their Lives, Times and Ideas* (New York: Times Books, 2000).

ACKNOWLEDGMENTS

IN 2012, when I completed *Forces of Change: New Strategies for the Evolving Health Care Marketplace*, I extended a tremendous debt of gratitude to those who contributed to the book. Upon its publication, I started envisioning *Launching and Leading Change Initiatives in Health Care Organizations* as an answer to the many requests for a book about my work in project management. I am so very fortunate to have had the same *Forces of Change* team intact for this new book. My thanks to Holly Zellweger of the Harvard School of Public Health, who was an invaluable contributor to editing and manuscript preparation, and in other countless ways. John Case has been a collaborator without peer. He is a consummate professional in regard to both form and substance.

My Jossey-Bass partners, the late Andy Pasternack, senior editor, and Seth Schwartz, associate editor, made this process pleasant and enriching. And thanks to draft manuscript reviewers Patricia Boer, Justin Or, Jennifer Wind, and Sumita Yadav for providing excellent suggestions and commentary.

To my wife, Charlotte, and children, Douglas and Alyssa, thank you for your support in all I do. I offer special recognition to Doug. As a young professional, he has made substantive contributions that were well beyond his years. I am unwavering in my belief that he will be an outstanding professional with project management skills and other assets from which every change initiative would benefit greatly.

Finally, I thank the students in my graduate course at Harvard. The curriculum from this course serves as the basis for this book. I also thank the professionals in my executive education programs from around the world who inspired me and encouraged me to write a book about how to launch successful projects.

DAVID A. SHORE

One of America's leading authorities on managing change initiatives and gaining a competitive advantage, David A. Shore, PhD, is a former associate dean of Harvard University's School of Public Health. During his two decades as a Harvard faculty member and executive director of the school's Center for Continuing Professional Education, Shore founded and directed the flagship executive programs Forces of Change: New Strategies for the Evolving Health Care Marketplace, the Trust Initiative, and the Certificate Program on Launching and Leading Successful Change Initiatives. The last of these programs is based on the Project Activation Management System (PAMS), which he developed.

He has served on and chaired numerous boards and committees, and currently sits on the board of directors of the Marshfield Clinic Health System as well as several editorial boards. A prolific author, his books include *The Trust Prescription for Healthcare: Building Your Reputation with Consumers; The Trust Crisis in Healthcare: Causes, Consequences, and Cures; High Stakes: The Critical Role of Stakeholders in Health Care* (with Eric D. Kupferberg); and *Forces of Change: New Strategies for the Evolving Health Care Marketplace.* Shore has been interviewed on various aspects of becoming a higher-performing organization in such publications as the *Wall Street Journal,* the *New York Times, INC,* and *Modern Healthcare.*

Prior to joining Harvard, Shore served in leadership roles at the Joint Commission, the Healthcare Financial Management Association, and the American College of Healthcare Executives.

Shore chaired the first, second, and third national Executive Conferences on Branding, Positioning, and Competitive Strategies. He has had the honor to deliver the keynote address for four annual Corporate Branding Conferences of the American Management Association. He chaired and delivered the keynote address at all three of the World Congress Leadership Summits on Project Management. He has consulted on six continents and has been selected to deliver more than one hundred named and keynote addresses throughout the world. Participants frequently comment that he brings his passion to the podium.

Shore is currently an adjunct professor of organizational development and change in the Business School, University of Monterrey, Mexico; lecturer at Harvard University Extension School; and a faculty member of The Governance Institute. He is also Executive in Residence at Enable East, a National Health Service team in the United Kingdom. He has held visiting professorships, including at the University of Amsterdam and IEDE Business School, Santiago, Chile.

Never known to simply "admire the problem," Shore is dedicated to building constructive links between theory and practice through his research, consulting, and educational endeavors. Shore provides executable advice, inspiring leaders and organizations to gain a unique and sustainable competitive advantage.

Launching and Leading Change Initiatives in Health Care Organizations

Changing Health Care

INTRODUCTION: THE NEED FOR CHANGE

As anyone who works in and around health care knows, it is an unusual environment. It is both a mission and an industry. It is a high-tech scientific enterprise and a high-touch human service. The overarching objective is simple enough, albeit often beyond our grasp: to help people recover from illnesses and injuries and stay healthy. But the subordinate goals are numerous and often in conflict. Health care organizations try to deliver care that is consistent with the best scientific evidence and that patients and their families also find helpful and comforting. They try to do so in a businesslike and cost-effective manner, so that their revenues exceed their expenses. (No margin, no mission, as the common phrase has it.) Perhaps most relevant for our purposes, they try to continually learn and improve, so that the care they offer tomorrow will be more effective, more helpful, and more efficient than the care they offer today. Change initiatives and projects are the route to organizational learning and improvement. They are the method by which people can make health care better.

There is little doubt that health care *needs* to get better.

Granted, U.S. health care in some respects is the best in the world. People from around the world often fly to the United States for treatment. Many Americans pronounce themselves satisfied with the care they receive. Still, the list of challenges is long, the failures persistent. U.S. health care is far more expensive than care in other countries, and the outcomes are often poorer. Costs continue to increase every year. Many people—close to half, according to one influential study—do not receive standard recommended care for their ailments.[1] Some failings seem almost intractable. "At least 44,000 people, and perhaps as many as 98,000 people, die in hospitals each year as a result of medical errors that could have been prevented," wrote the Institute of Medicine in its landmark 1999 report.[2] The numbers have been debated—some think the record is worse—but no one is arguing that things have improved much since then.

The amount of waste in health care is another of those seemingly intractable problems, and one that is particularly germane to the subject of this book. Data from various studies indicate that about 30 percent of health care spending in the United States is wasteful, in the sense that it does not improve health. This represents about $750 billion in annual expenditures, or more than 5 percent of U.S. gross domestic product. Waste comes in many forms, and several different studies have tried to categorize them. Donald Berwick and Andrew Hackbarth, for example, have identified six major categories of waste: failures of care delivery, failures of care coordination, overtreatment, administrative complexity, pricing failures, and fraud and abuse.[3] The omnipresent business meeting in health care organizations is both a symptom and a cause of waste. For example, a community hospital affiliated with a medical school in the western United States holds a monthly one-hour meeting for its 110-plus managers and supervisors. Many attendees gain little from this meeting; in fact, a significant number of people admit to "dreading" it. Yet every single meeting costs the hospital at least $11,660 in direct costs—the time of the participants—and untold thousands more in opportunity costs. One might ask why the hospital leadership isn't dreading spending so much on this meeting each month. Why are they embracing the meeting that so many of its participants dread?[4]

The contradictions in the health care system—care that is often superb juxtaposed with skyrocketing costs, countless errors, and enormous waste—are reflected in what people on the front lines see and hear every day. On the one hand, it seems that everyone is talking about change. Executives and administrators issue pronouncements on the need to improve. Organizations launch initiative after initiative. New laws, new technologies, and rising consumer expectations all push institutions to improve the way they operate. On the other hand, lasting change seems hard to come by. Initiatives fail. Clinicians and other health care workers continue behaving today much as they did yesterday and the day before that. Not long ago, the Harvard School of Public Health and the consulting firm Towers Watson joined forces to conduct a survey, asking hospital CEOs and other senior administrators about their efforts to change. "There remains what we would call a 'say/do gap' in how hospitals currently address and implement new initiatives," the study concluded. "The hospital executives who responded to our survey said they understood the steps essential to successful project implementation. But they also acknowledged that their organization's follow-through on some of these steps is inconsistent at best."[5] If a visitor from Mars were to assess hospitals and other health care organizations, he or she might conclude that they all want to get better—indeed, to be the best in their class. They just do not want to change.

There are reasons for this reluctance. Health care has many stakeholders, and it is a rare occasion indeed when all of them share the same interest in change. A reform that one group supports may be adamantly opposed by other groups. What one stakeholder views as an elimination of waste may be seen by another stakeholder as an assault on his or her income or prestige. Then, too, medicine as an enterprise is necessarily conservative. "First, do no harm" is still a time-honored precept, as it should be. Clinicians rightly want to know that a proposed change really will do no harm, and that the chances that it will lead to better outcomes are high. Of course, this conservative attitude can be, and often is, taken to a harmful extreme. One unit of a health care organization may mistrust the motives of another, and so refuse to have anything to do with a change that the other unit proposes. And all organizations have their share of what I call CAVE people—those who are Constantly Against Virtually Everything.

But these aren't the only reasons for health care's failure to change. There has also been a chronic deficiency in leadership and vision. Most health care organizations do not go about change in the right way. They start things they never finish. Sometimes they get bogged down in details when they should be looking at the big picture; other times they focus on a vision of the future while ignoring the messy details of reality. Most important for our purposes, they pay too little attention to the launching of an initiative, and then are surprised when it never takes off. They are like a pilot who assumes the plane is airborne before it ever leaves the ground.

What nearly every health care organization I have seen needs, and often lacks, is a deep understanding of how hard the *process* of change really is, and how the difficulties can be eased by a systematic approach. That is the subject of this part of the book. We will look closely at the process and see what is required to address it. We will examine what it means for an initiative to succeed, and how good planning can put it on the path to success. Along the way, I hope, you will begin to understand how to create that systematic approach to change that really can begin to improve health care.

SUMMARY

- Despite its accomplishments, U.S. health care faces significant challenges.

- Most health care organizations have many projects under way, but few organizations have been successful in actually changing the way they operate.

- The chief reason for this failure is the absence of a systematic approach to change.

NOTES

1. Elizabeth A. McGlynn et al., "The Quality of Health Care Delivered to Adults in the United States," *New England Journal of Medicine* 348 (2003): 2635–2645.
2. Institute of Medicine, *To Err Is Human: Building a Safer Health System* (Washington, DC: National Academies Press, November 1999), http://www.iom.edu/~/media/Files/Report%20Files/1999/To-Err-is-Human/To%20Err%20is%20Human%201999%20%20report%20brief.pdf.
3. Donald M. Berwick and Andrew D. Hackbarth, "Eliminating Waste in U.S. Health Care," *Journal of the American Medical Association* 307 (2012): 1513–1516.
4. See David A. Shore, with Douglas A. Shore, "From 'Wasteful' Meetings to Parsimonious Meetings Management: Preserving Human Capital in Health Care Delivery Organizations" (working paper, Harvard School of Public Health, Boston, April 2013). Available from the senior author at shoredavida@gmail.com.
5. David A. Shore et al., *The Hospital Industry in Transition: Building Capability to Successfully Drive Change* (Harvard School of Public Health, Towers Watson, 2011), 4, http://www.towerswatson.com/DownloadMedia.aspx?media=%7BCF62E9B2–2195–4DDC-BE75-FA9730B8282A%7D.

1

How Organizations Can *Really* Change

Leon C. Megginson (inspired by Charles Darwin) said that it is not the strongest of the species that survives, nor the most intelligent, but the one most responsive to change.[1]

General Erik Shinseki, who was U.S. Army chief of staff from 1999 to 2003, said, "If you don't like change, you will like irrelevance even less."[2]

The quality guru W. Edwards Deming put the matter even more starkly: "It is not necessary to change. Survival is not mandatory."[3]

Though health care offers few guarantees, there may be one simple truth that everyone in the field can agree on. Organizations that embrace change will stand the best chance of surviving, prospering, and delivering better care. Those that shrink from change are likely to be put out of business, or else be swallowed up by more nimble competitors.

Change, of course, is a loaded word, fraught with emotion and associations.

High up in the organization, few question its desirability. Chief executives and their senior management teams typically want to be known as bold, forward looking, visionary. They may assume that the need for change is equally visible to everyone, from the boardroom to the operating room to the kitchen—or that it soon will be, once the leaders explain it to everybody. Some leaders seem to think that change will happen automatically; all they have to do is announce the goal and the timeline.

This affection for bold reforms and visionary improvements is why "change talk" seems to permeate so many health care organizations. But what is the reaction to all the talk once you leave the C-suites and move out into the finance office or obstetrics ward? In my experience, people welcome change about as enthusiastically as they would welcome a plague of locusts. *Watch out*, the feeling runs. *Here comes another one. Maybe if you keep your head down it will go away.* Buddhists say that we are frightened by new things, and so we experience the suffering of change. The reason for this fear and loathing is that change always involves giving something up. We lose what we know in return for a promise of an uncertain future. People may even greet change with a kind of grief reaction, exhibiting all the familiar stages we have learned from Elisabeth Kübler-Ross.[4] *Denial*: Confronted by change, we confidently assert that it isn't really going to happen. *Anger*: We get mad. ("They can't do this to *me!*") *Depression*: We feel sad, demoralized. *Bargaining*: We negotiate to keep a little of what we had before. Sometimes I think that people faced with change undergo all the stages of grief except the last one, *acceptance*.

Change, in short, makes everybody uncomfortable. Like the body's homeostatic system, the mind naturally reverts to the familiar, the well-worn, the time-tested and trusted patterns of behavior. The mental system returns to its comfort zone. This is why change is so hard, and why so many change events or initiatives peter out, unsuccessful. The all-too-frequent approach from senior management—"Of course you will want to buy into the change I am proposing"—leaves people not only uninspired but anxious as well. It is little wonder that health care organizations, where every employee typically has plenty on his or her mind anyway, find it so difficult to do anything differently. Most stakeholders seem to view a proposed change skeptically, and the proposal stalls before it can get out of the starting gate.

A BETTER APPROACH

But let us imagine that you are a health care leader who actually wants change to *happen*, rather than simply to be announced. Let us imagine you are prepared to follow through, to mount the kind of systematic attack on the status quo that this book will prepare you for. The first thing you will need is a different mind-set, one that in some ways has been alien to health care. You will have to acknowledge difficult truths and use a different vocabulary. You will have to borrow from other industries. You will have to adopt some elements of marketing, often seen as anathema by medical professionals. Action is essential, of course, and the rest of this book will describe the actions necessary to get your change initiatives off to a productive start. But first must come the thoughts, assumptions, and attitudes that will inform your actions. Today's health care leaders must embrace five key changes in their attitudes.

1. Acknowledge How Hard Change Can Be

Nobody should ever assume that change will come easily. We all know from experience how difficult it is for anyone to change even minor aspects of his or her behavior. How many times have we made a New Year's resolution to alter our eating habits or visit the gym regularly, only to find ourselves making the identical resolution the following year? Despite such knowledge, we somehow seem to assume that change will come more readily to organizations. It will not. Organizations, after all, are just collections of individuals pursuing various sets of objectives. Training, expectations, habit, and inertia govern how they go about this pursuit. If people are to behave differently, they will need new training and new sets of expectations, and they will need to develop new habits and a new baseline of action. All of that requires a considerable amount of time and a lot of effort. Progress will be uneven—two steps forward, one step back. Organizations have a built-in resistance to change, and to ignore that fact is to set yourself up for failure.

So don't ignore it. Accompany every change initiative you propose with a deep understanding that this will mean loss for some people. Acknowledge that you will meet resistance, and that resistance is perfectly normal, even healthy. Sit down and assess the risks you face in advance. (The history of your organization's past change efforts is often a good guide to the difficulties you will encounter in the future.) Develop tools for mitigating those risks. Involve the people who will be affected in creating the change you want to see. Adopting this perspective will lend credibility to your efforts, and it will build trust. Nobody believes a leader who says change will be easy.

2. Accept and Communicate the Idea That, Whatever the Difficulties, Change Is Not Optional

It is a funny thing. In nearly every other industry these days, sentiments like those with which I began this chapter adorn the walls. They appear in executives' speeches. They are so common as to be commonplace. *Of course* change is not optional. *Of course* we must adapt or die. Nearly every other industry is littered with the remnants of companies that were once strong competitors but, challenged by their resistance to change, at some point suddenly ceased to exist. Think TWA or Pan Am, Polaroid or RCA, Netscape or Atari. (Some of these brands live on, but the companies themselves are long gone.) However, few health care organizations make the same assumptions. They may talk about reforms and improvements, but they rarely assume that change is an imperative. They may say, "Innovate or die," but they do not act as if they believe it.

A few organizations, however—generally the highest performers— embrace a wholly different way of thinking, known as *permanent beta.*

Beta is a term borrowed from the technology world, where it refers to products that are still in testing and hence not quite finished. Successful organizations realize that they are never perfect, and that virtually everything about them can always be improved. They exist in a state of permanent beta. Not only do they *exist* in a state of permanent beta, but also they regularly *talk* about being in a state of permanent beta. "Words are like children," said Martin Luther in a 2003 biopic. "The more attention we pay to them, the more demanding they become."[5] When you use words like *permanent beta* regularly, they worm their way into people's consciousness. They become a part of the organizational culture. They encourage the idea that change is never-ending—that it is not an "event" that happens at a single point in time. The expectation of change becomes a part of people's daily work lives.

3. Embrace "From—To"

Every change event attempts to move an organization *from* a current state *to* a future state. That is why so many people greet the effort with skepticism at best and hostility at worst. "You want me to leave my safe, secure, familiar, comfortable world in exchange for—what? A brave new world that you *say* will be better? Are you crazy?" Health care professionals and staff in particular are rarely excited about moving from their present state to some future state. Health care has been a growing industry. Most organizations are doing well enough, and many individuals within those organizations are busy, well paid, and highly satisfied with their respective jobs. The changes mandated by new government policies such as the Patient Protection and Affordable Care Act threaten to upset a lot of these applecarts. So clinicians and others in health care have a strong inclination to leave well enough alone. "If it ain't broke, don't fix it." Even seemingly unexceptionable goals, such as pursuing evidence-based medicine and embracing electronic health records, often run into massive resistance.

But what if today's world is no longer so safe and comfortable? What if people in an organization learn, through constant repetition, that the status quo is unpleasant, unsafe, uncomfortable, and above all unstable? Health care costs have been rising steadily and inexorably. There has been *no* improvement in the rate of amenable mortality. The health care system wastes 30 percent of its resources. "If you think this situation can continue forever," a leader might say, "you are living in a dream world. If we fail to change, one of two things will happen. One possibility is that we will be forced to change, on somebody else's timetable, by government edict or insurance company policy or in response to the expectations of the marketplace. The other possibility is that we will have no opportunity to change, because we will have been forced out of business."

This kind of thinking—making people uncomfortable with the current state of affairs—alters the terms of the equation. Marketers have known this for centuries, and have used it effectively. "Your clothes are drab, your car is unexciting, your medicine doesn't make you feel better, your cooking is terrible. But all you have to do is buy our product, and that will solve your problem." I am not suggesting that health care leaders turn themselves into full-time marketers. I am suggesting that they learn the basic psychology that underlies marketing: people will not change unless they feel dissatisfied with the current situation. Other businesses talk about creating "burning platforms." People will be receptive to new ideas when they feel that their platform really is burning.

4. Think *Kaizen*

Here is another example of how far health care lags behind most other industries in its approach to change. The Japanese word *kaizen*, which essentially means "change for the better" or "continuous improvement," is now used regularly on factory floors in America. Plant managers and employees have come to understand that it is their responsibility, every day and every week, to call out and address the little things that go wrong, the inefficiencies, the bottlenecks, the ways of operating that might have once made sense but no longer do. Some plants sponsor kaizen events, in which employees take time off from their regular work to identify dozens or hundreds of potential improvements, evaluate them, and implement as many as possible.

Kaizen as a concept has made only limited inroads in health care. But health care as an industry probably has more inefficiencies, bottlenecks, and unnecessary procedures than manufacturing ever did. Kaizen is simply a way of helping people identify those glitches and take steps to eliminate them. In health care organizations, it is often very effective to bring stakeholders together and solicit suggestions to improve a challenging issue. I refer to this process as a kaizen town hall meeting.

5. Understand the Psychological Factors That Affect People's Perceptions

We human beings are peculiar animals. We have an extremely well-developed cerebral cortex, and we think a great deal of it. We value intelligence, rationality, and deliberation. Yet when we make decisions, we are affected by emotional factors of which we are scarcely aware. Again, marketers understand this phenomenon well. They tell stories as well as make arguments. They present us with appealing images, not just words. They understand that we are hardwired to make decisions with emotions first and thoughts second. They appeal to head and heart simultaneously, but the appeal to the heart usually takes precedence.

This emotions-first approach to decision making has two ramifications. One is that people tend to prefer the specific over the general. We ignore a headline about a devastating earthquake somewhere in the world, but we reach for the telephone when an aid organization shows us some of its suffering victims up close and personal.[6] The other is that we fear loss more than we value an equal gain. This is the cognitive bias known as loss aversion, and it has been demonstrated repeatedly in a series of experiments.[7] Where change is concerned, the uncertainty surrounding the future state of affairs is thus likely to outweigh whatever benefits we think we may get from it. We overestimate the value of what we have and underestimate the value of what may be gained by giving it up.

Health care leaders can put this understanding of human psychology to work in the way they frame proposals for change. To get true buy-in, they can appeal jointly to head and heart: no statistic without a story, no story without a statistic, as the axiom of persuasion has it. They can help people visualize and imagine the future state so that everyone begins to *feel* its desirability. They cannot ignore the necessary losses that always accompany change; attempting to do so costs them their credibility and undermines trust. But they can help people remember the losses, such as a potential threat to job security, that will inevitably accompany a *failure* to change. Those losses are presumably far more significant than anything the change itself is likely to bring.

Will there be resistance? Of course. Everybody knows that nobody likes change except a wet baby. Resistance is a healthy sign, a sign that people are taking the prospect of change seriously. They will be anxious, uncertain, skeptical. But a positive approach to managing change can help people work through their resistance and come out on the other side.

FROM "PROJECTS" TO CHANGE EVENTS

These five changes in the leader's attitudes are essential. They can help people in an organization overcome their natural uncertainty about doing things differently. But by themselves they are insufficient. Leaders also need to create a new way of thinking about the process of change. If there were a mantra for this part of the book, it would be, "Don't leave change to chance."

To begin, it is worth remembering that change itself can be systematically analyzed and codified, and many leading thinkers have done so. The classic 1951 book by the social psychologist Kurt Lewin described the three phases of change as "unfreeze," "transition," and "refreeze."[8] This cycle can be repeated as necessary. Lewin's phases are intuitive to most and serve as a basic foundation for conceptualizing change in an organization. Harvard Business School professor John Kotter has outlined an eight-stage process for creating major change:[9]

1. Establishing a sense of urgency

2. Creating the guiding coalition

3. Developing a vision and strategy

4. Communicating the change vision

5. Empowering broad-based action

6. Generating short-term wins

7. Consolidating gains and producing more change

8. Anchoring new approaches in the culture

Note that some of Kotter's stages involve the kind of marketing mind-set we have just been discussing—establishing a sense of urgency, communicating the change vision, and so on. But others have to do with the mechanics of actually creating change and embedding it in the way the organization goes about its business—such as empowering broad-based action and anchoring new approaches in the culture.

Change can even be encapsulated in equations, which help us remember the key variables and the interactions between them. For example, a well-known formulation by organizational development specialists Richard Beckhard and Reuben Harris (refined by Kathie Dannemiller) looks like this:[10]

$$D \times V \times F > R$$

where
D = Dissatisfaction
V = Vision
F = First steps
R = Resistance to change

The formula can be used as a diagnostic aid to determine whether an organization is ready for change. All three components—dissatisfaction with the current situation, a vision of what is possible in the future, and achievable first steps toward reaching this vision—must be present if the organization is to overcome its resistance to change. The formula helps answer the question, "Can we successfully undertake change? Are our people and our organization prepared?"

Another useful equation is this one, used by the company GE Healthcare:[11]

$$E = Q \times A^3$$

where
E = Effective results
Q = Quality of the solution
A = Acceptance of the idea
A = Alignment with organizational goals
A = Accountability for the implementation

Some 62 percent of change efforts fail, says the company, due to lack of attention to the "A"—really, the multiple "A's"—in the equation. You don't get good results unless the change effort fits the organization and people are held accountable for implementing it successfully.

Many large organizations, including some in health care, have attempted to systematize their approach to change by creating a project management office (PMO). The office is responsible for overseeing, managing, and evaluating the initiatives through which the organization hopes to change and improve. This is a step in the right direction, and later chapters will discuss some of the functions such an office can perform as well as variations on the theme.

But for now, let's just look at the language. The word *project* suggests a nuts-and-bolts engineering enterprise. The phrase *project management* conjures up visions of workers in hard hats on a construction site. Make no mistake: projects are worthy endeavors, and I will sometimes use that language in this book just because it is so common. But *change* is broader, more inspiring, and ultimately more accurate in describing what needs to happen in health care. Suppose we thought of every project as a change event, every project manager as an agent of change, and the PMO as a change office. Change is scary, to be sure. But properly managed—with the mind-set I have outlined in this chapter—it can be inspiring, exciting, even thrilling. A project operates in a business-as-usual context, and is content to make a small improvement in everyday operations. A change event is part of a movement toward a goal, a step toward realizing the organization's mission. It can be approached every bit as systematically as a project, and managed just as intensively. But it is a goal that is worth the effort, a journey that can get people fired up and wanting to climb on board.

Indeed, project-based work is steadily growing. It is becoming more common for colleagues to band together as a change initiative team to undertake a prescribed piece of work. Once the task is completed, the team disbands, only to be reorganized into new teams for new change events.

I don't mean to load too much onto the backs of mere words. You will read about managing projects as well as about managing change in this book. If you modify the language you use to describe change without modifying the reality, you will not be making much of a difference. But words do matter, as does context. Right now, health care needs a mind-set that welcomes change; that acknowledges its difficulties; and that embraces the paths leading to real, sustainable change. That is an enterprise worthy of a true leader, and one that I believe will be the hallmark of higher-performing organizations.

SUMMARY

- "Change talk" permeates most health care organizations, but real change is seldom welcomed at all levels of an organization.

- Leaders need to adopt a different mind-set—acknowledging how hard change is, understanding that it is not optional, and making people uncomfortable with the current state of affairs.

- Leaders also need to borrow from other industries, drawing on the concept of *kaizen* (continuous improvement) and the tools of marketing, which appeal to people's emotions as well as their intellect.

- Don't leave change to chance. Look at it systematically, and build enthusiasm for change events.

NOTES

1. Leon C. Megginson, "Lessons from Europe for American Business," *Southwestern Social Science Quarterly* 44, no. 1 (1963): 4.
2. Fast Company, *The Rules of Business: 55 Essential Ideas to Help Smart People (and Organizations) Perform at Their Best* (New York: Crown Business, 2005), 7.
3. Attributed to W. Edwards Deming at "W. Edwards Deming quotes," accessed April 29, 2013, http://en.thinkexist.com/quotes/w._edwards_deming/2.html.
4. Elisabeth Kübler-Ross, *On Death and Dying* (New York: Macmillan, 1969).
5. "Luther Script—Dialogue Transcript," accessed April 29, 2013, http://www.script-o-rama.com/movie_scripts/l/luther-script-transcript-joseph-fiennes.html.
6. See, for example, Deborah A. Small, George Loewenstein, and Paul Slovic, "Sympathy and Callousness: The Impact of Deliberative Thought on Donations to Identifiable and Statistical Victims," *Organizational Behavior and Human Decision Processes* 102, no. 2 (March 2007): 143–153.
7. Daniel Kahneman, Jack Knetsch, and Richard Thaler, "Experimental Test of the Endowment Effect and the Coase Theorem," *Journal of Political Economy* 98, no. 6 (1990): 1325–1348; Amos Tversky and Daniel Kahneman, "Loss Aversion in

Riskless Choice: A Reference Dependent Model," *Quarterly Journal of Economics* 106 (1991): 1039–1061; Daniel Kahneman, Jack Knetsch, and Richard Thaler, "Anomalies: The Endowment Effect, Loss Aversion, and Status Quo Bias," *Journal of Economic Perspectives* 5, no. 1 (Winter 1991): 193–206.

8. Kurt Lewin, *Field Theory in Social Science* (New York: Harper & Row, 1951).

9. Adapted from John P. Kotter, "Why Transformation Efforts Fail," *Harvard Business Review* 73, no. 2 (March–April 1995): 59–67.

10. Cited in Dannemiller Tyson Associates, *Whole-Scale Change: Unleashing the Magic in Organizations* (San Francisco: Berrett-Koehler, 2000), 16.

11. Justin Holland, *Prescription for Effective Change* (Waukesha, WI: GE Healthcare, 2011), 7, http://nextlevel.gehealthcare.com/Prescription_For_Effective_Change-WP-0811.pdf.

2

Criteria for an Initiative's Success

Every change initiative begins with high hopes. "It will improve the care we offer patients. It will make for better outcomes. It will make us more efficient, lower our costs, save time." And indeed: why should this not be the case? Projects or initiatives are a catalyst for change. They are the method for moving *from* the current state of affairs *to* a better future. They are the vehicle to carry an idea from concept to reality. They are the way health care organizations innovate and thus improve. John F. Kennedy is thought to have said that the only reason to give a speech is to change the world. Initiatives by definition are about changing the world—the world of health care. That is their justification, their reason for being. No wonder they are launched with such grand aspirations.

And yet every project is fraught with risk. It is an experiment, the outcome of which is uncertain. No one can ever say that a particular project is going to work as originally envisioned. Project team members know—or should know—that the best they can do is try to make things better. They also know that there will be a heavy price to pay if they inadvertently make things worse. As I noted in chapter 1, health care is an unforgiving context for change initiatives. A failed project can lead to poorer medical outcomes, even increased mortality, as well as less efficiency or effectiveness in an organization's operations.

Given these homely truths, it is worth looking at the record of failure before we consider the criteria for success.

FAILURE RATES

A management consultant named Ivars Avots, who worked for the firm Arthur D. Little, once summed up his studies of project success and failure. "The many instances where project management fails," Avots wrote, "overshadow the stories of successful projects."[1] His conclusion might hardly be worth mentioning except for three things. One, the author was a noted expert in the field of management. Two, he published the study in 1969. Three, little has changed in the past forty-plus years in regard to success rates.

Look, for example, at studies of IT (information technology) projects, which are just one kind of initiative health care organizations undertake and which in some ways are among the easiest to accomplish (table 2.1). Success rates ranged between 26 percent and 35 percent. Close to half of the projects were "challenged"—that is, they may have been completed, but

Table 2.1 Project Resolution History

	2000	2002	2004	2006	2008	2010
Succeeded	28%	34%	29%	35%	32%	37%
Challenged	49%	51%	53%	46%	44%	42%
Failed	23%	15%	18%	19%	24%	21%

Source: Data from the Standish Group, *CHAOS Manifesto* (2010), 5, and the Standish Group, *The True Cost of a Project* (2012), 1, https://secure.standishgroup.com/reports/reports.php.

they took too long, ran over budget, or offered fewer features and functions than originally planned. The rest were outright failures. Worst of all, there was no trend toward improvement: 2008 was worse than the years immediately preceding it. As lawyers say, *res ipsa loquitur*: the facts speak for themselves. We are not getting any better.

What about data for health care projects in general? What I have found is that very few organizations even track their failure rates. Their managers and employees have no idea what the rates might be. Yet if you do not know your failure rates, you cannot learn why projects are failing, and you cannot improve your rates of success. It is hard to prevent failure when you cannot even grasp the magnitude of the problem.

The lack of data is symptomatic of another ailment as well. Health care projects fail in many different ways, some of them quite subtle. They slowly peter out. They achieve part of their objectives and are abandoned. They meet their goals in one area but fail to meet their goals in another. Most insidious, *no one really knows how well the project did.* Just as it is rare to find an organization that tracks its failure rates, it is rare to find one that has even defined failure. These of course are two sides of the same coin. You can't accurately track failure unless you know what it is. Ask yourself whether your organization has a project monitoring system. Does it identify and mitigate projects that find themselves in trouble? If the answer to these questions is no, you are flying blind. You do not know where you are going off track, so you cannot know how to get back on track.

In chapter 3 we will examine some ways to "fail better." But our first task is to understand what it means to fail, which necessarily involves understanding the criteria for success.

DOING THE RIGHT THING RIGHT

Every initiative can be judged on two dimensions. First, is it the right thing to be doing? Second, is the organization going about it in the right way?

Put these two criteria together, and you come up with what might be called an accuracy/quality matrix, in which accuracy refers to undertaking the right projects and quality refers to doing things right (figure 2.1). If

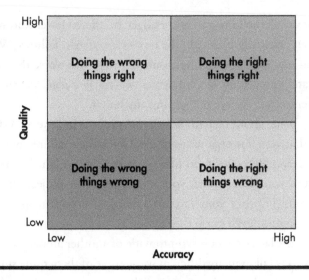

Figure 2.1 Project Accuracy/Quality Matrix

Source: Adapted from Chuck Musciano, "Right or Wrong? Well or Poorly?" *The Effective CIO* (blog), March 9, 2009, http://effectivecio.com/2009/03/02/rght-or-wrong-well-or-poorly/.

this book were printed in color, the lower left-hand corner of the matrix would be bright red, the color of a stoplight. Nobody wants to do the wrong things wrong. The upper-left and lower-right quadrants might be yellow: something isn't the way it ought to be. Only the upper-right quadrant would be green, indicating full speed ahead.

This is a terribly simple gauge of projects, and yet we need simplicity at this stage. The reason we need such a matrix is that health care is notorious for practices and projects that land squarely in one of those yellow quadrants. Consider the phenomenon of wrong-site surgeries—doing the wrong thing right. In 2004 the Joint Commission began requiring physicians and nurses to follow a universal protocol as a way of eliminating wrong-site surgeries. Before every operation, hospital personnel were supposed to verify and mark the part of the body to be operated on. Surgical staff were expected to take a time-out immediately before the operation to ensure that they were working on the correct part. Yet wrong-site surgeries continue to happen as often as forty times a week, according to Joint Commission estimates in 2011. "In two states that track and intensively study these errors," the *Washington Post* reported, "48 cases were reported in Minnesota last year, up from 44 in 2009; Pennsylvania has averaged about 64 cases for the past few years." Recent incidents in other states included an ophthalmologist operating on the wrong eye of a four-year-old, and three wrong-site spinal surgeries in two months at a Boston hospital.[2]

There are many other examples of doing the wrong thing right, albeit not quite so gruesome. A hospital builds a sparkling new wing and finds that it can't fill the beds, because other hospitals in the region have been adding capacity as well. A physician practice installs a top-of-the-line system for maintaining electronic health records and then learns that the new system is incompatible with the ancient IT system at the doctors' primary hospital.

Doing the right thing wrong is unfortunately all too common. Hospitals and pharmacies dispense the wrong medication, often (still!) because dispensing pharmacists cannot read physicians' handwriting. Hospitals and physicians submit improperly coded bills to insurance companies, and the insurance companies then refuse payment. Often both factors— quality and accuracy—are involved when a project fails to meet its objectives. Consider the following example from a report on the hospital industry that I collaborated on with the consulting firm Towers Watson: "One hospital...completed a major remodeling of its bathrooms to comply with the requirements of the Americans with Disabilities Act. However, the engineering team didn't involve the occupational therapists working with the patients. As a result, the team installed expensive wall-mounted shower benches that were not adjustable and were virtually unusable for patients recovering from hip replacements and other surgeries. Had the therapists been consulted, they would have recommended a less expensive and labor-intensive option that would have met needs far more effectively."[3] The project team in this case went about its work in the wrong way and thereby ended up doing the wrong thing.

Every industry faces this fundamental set of constraints, whatever it does. A direct-mail marketer might be a whiz at designing appealing promotional packages. If he is trying to sell snowblowers in Florida, however, he is doing the wrong thing right. Health care is no exception. The "right thing" is whatever improves the lives of a given set of stakeholders in a way that is consistent with the organization's mission, vision, and values. The right methodology actually helps achieve this objective.

APPROPRIATE MEASURES OF SUCCESS

The word *right*, of course, is one that is subject to interpretation. You might say that rightness, like beauty, is in the eye of the beholder. *Wrong* is easy to identify, but right is hard. Only when it is attached to specifications and measurements does it have a well-defined meaning.

Projects traditionally have been gauged by three fundamental measures.

The first measure is *scope*—the work to be performed. Scope defines exactly what the project is supposed to accomplish. By implication, it also defines what is *not* included in the project. Scope creep, of course, is common. A project that starts out to achieve one set of results may find that it has many more objectives added on to it before it is complete. Because a project's scope is mapped out in advance, success on this dimension can be gauged at any point in time partly by whether the project is reaching its objectives.

The second measure is *cost*, or budget. The budget defines the resources available for the project. A project performed by an outside vendor typically has a fixed budget defined by a contract, though even fixed budgets are known sometimes to increase. Projects performed in-house may or may not have a formal budget attached to them. If they do, the budget may creep upward just as the scope does. (The two are related.) A project that is on budget is meeting another test of success.

The third measure is *time*, or the schedule for the project. Everybody dreads deadlines, but nobody can avoid them entirely. Even projects that stretch their initial timeline have to end someday. Or at least they should. A project that is successful will be completed on time.

These are the ubiquitous gauges of projects, the tendons that hold them together. Each one affects the other. An upward-creeping scope is likely to cost more and take longer. Reducing the time frame may compromise the scope. As chief financial officers like to say, you can have it good, fast, or cheap—pick two. Joking aside, the most common definition of an initiative's success is that it comes in on time, on budget, and to specification.

But although these three metrics of success may be enough for some industries, they are not adequate for health care. They are necessary but not sufficient. They are myopic and internally focused. They judge the project purely on its own terms. They remind one of the old saw in medicine, "The operation was a success, but the patient died." The equivalent in project terms might be, "The project came in on spec, on budget, and on time—and it made things worse."

What might more appropriate measures of success look like? I typically consider three.

One is that the project *stays live*. Here's why: By definition, a project has a precise beginning and a precise end. When the project is completed, the end result is handed off to an operations team. It is the operations team's responsibility to maintain the end result and make sure it "stays live." In the world of projects and initiatives, team members always focus on the day that the project will "go live." That's when the work will be done, the project will be turned into a process, and the change will take effect. But we need to ask what is happening three months, six months, or twelve months later. It makes no difference whether the project met the three traditional measures of success if its impact fades away or it disappears entirely.

A second measure might be that the project *is fit for use*. A successful project gains the approval of the people it affects because it somehow makes their work easier, more efficient, or more effective. It meets its stakeholders' needs. Imagine the installation of a new financial management system. The system may be up and running on time and on budget—but what if in practice it turns out to be a clunker, harder to use than the one it replaced? Or imagine designing and implementing a new protocol to reduce infections in intensive care units. The project might be executed perfectly yet fail to achieve the desired result because the chief sources of infections lie outside its scope. Failure to consider fitness for use often leads to failure of the project.

The third measure requires a section all its own, because in health care little is as important as this gauge: the project *limits the risk involved* only to what is required. It exposes no one to unnecessary risk, and it manages necessary risk appropriately. Let's look at what this entails.

CAREFUL MANAGEMENT OF RISK

"Great deeds are usually wrought at great risk," wrote the Greek historian Herodotus. In health care, however, even modest deeds can entail substantial risks, for the reasons I have already enumerated. The prime virtue of the status quo in any health care setting is that it usually works reasonably well. A change initiative or project threatens to upend the status quo. It promises to reshape some processes, abolish others, create completely new ones, or do all of the above. So risk is built in from the beginning. The nature of the environment tends to compound the risk. We can think of projects as being either *linear*—one step following another in an observable, well-defined sequence, as on an assembly line—or *nonlinear*, characterized by independent and opaque interactions that are usually unpredictable (think of the global economy). Projects in health care may start out linear, in the sense that a project team maps out a series of sequential steps. But they nearly always wind up nonlinear because the environment changes so rapidly. Because projects are experiments, we really can't say for sure that they are going to unfold as envisioned. And, not surprisingly, the greater the nonlinearity, the greater the risk.

What are the sources of risk? Some sources are external—a change in government regulations, for instance, or a change in the price of necessary equipment while the project is under way. Others are internal to the organization. For example, an organization may acquire another organization or itself be acquired. It may redirect its strategic focus, so that what seemed important yesterday is no longer important today. And still others are internal to the project team itself. Team members may be ignorant of some factor or variable that will turn out to be important. Or they may do their jobs improperly. In general, risk varies with three factors: the size and

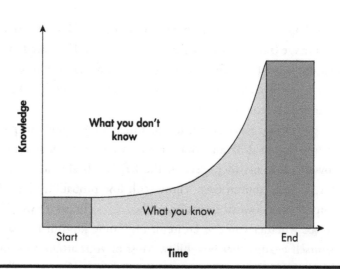

Figure 2.2 The Knowledge Curve

Source: Randall L. Englund, *Project Sponsorship: Achieving Management Commitment for Project Success* (San Francisco: Jossey-Bass, 2006), 54.

nature of a project, the amount of change involved, and the level of project management experience in an organization.[4]

Whatever the source, risk is likely to decline over time. At the beginning of a project, nobody knows how it is going to turn out. As the project proceeds, everyone gains a good deal more knowledge (figure 2.2). The uncertainty—and the chances of something going wrong—thus diminish.

Because the uncertainty is so high at the beginning, the identification and management of risk are essential to project success. Let's look at some techniques.

Risk is by definition an event that may occur in the future. A change initiative team can identify the most likely risks and then quantify them in a two-step process. First, the team asks what the probability is that a given event will occur. Probabilities, of course, range from 0 to 100 percent. Then the team asks, if the event does occur, how large of an impact will it have, again on a scale from 0 to 100 percent? The two figures together indicate the magnitude of the risk. Imagine that you are planning your daughter's wedding. Depending on where you live and the time of year, the risk of rain will range (say) from 10 percent to 90 percent. If the wedding is to be held outdoors, with no tent, the impact of a rainy day could be considerable. If it is to be held indoors, the impact would be negligible. To judge the risk, you need to consider both factors.

With key risks quantified in this manner, you can plot them on a graph (figure 2.3) and draw bands separating them into clusters. The lower-risk items (depicted on the left band) should go on a watch list for periodic monitoring. Those with low probability but high potential impact may devastate a project if they do occur, so it's worth investigating to see whether you can create or buy some kind of insurance to protect yourself against that possibility. Most of your attention should go to the high-probability, high-impact risks that you have identified, which are depicted in the upper-right area of the right band. That is where you will want to focus your risk management and risk mitigation efforts.

Project teams need to ask two additional questions about potential risk factors. At what point in the initiative's life cycle is the event likely to affect

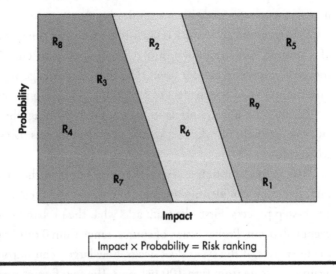

Figure 2.3   Risk Probability and Impact Matrix

Source: Adapted from Project Management Institute, *A Guide to the Project Management Body of Knowledge: PMBOK* (Newtown Square, PA: Project Management Institute, 2008).

the project? And how often is the event likely to occur? Both of these also affect prioritization in risk management. The ramifications of frequency are obvious. As for timing, the impact of a risk event is less if it occurs earlier rather than later, because the project can more easily adapt. It is obviously simpler and cheaper to alter a new IT system when the system is still in the design stage than it is once the hardware and software have been installed. Indeed, for any project, the pain of changing something is far lower when the project is in the development stage.

With risk factors identified and quantified, you can adopt strategies of managing and mitigating risk. The goal is to minimize risks wherever possible and mitigate the effects of risk events should they occur. There are four basic approaches:

- **Avoid the risk.** In other words, create a prevention plan. Figure out what you need to do to ensure that the event in question doesn't occur.

- **Transfer the risk.** Buy insurance. Make it somebody else's job to worry about that risk.

- **Mitigate the risk.** Create a plan for handling the effects of the risk event and reducing its likely impact.

- **Accept the risk.** Realize that some risks cannot be avoided, transferred, or mitigated, and that all you can do is create a contingency plan or work-around for dealing with it when and if it occurs.

Because there is so much to watch out for in many projects, it nearly always makes sense to designate one team member as the official risk watcher. He or she will be charged, among other things, with monitoring the risks as the project progresses, updating the evaluations, and keeping other project members informed on how the risk profile of the project is evolving. I will come back to this idea later in the book.

The single greatest contributor to a lack of control in projects is failure to consider and deal with risk. And the single greatest risk-mitigating strategy is to proceed slowly, step by step, learning by testing and doing and then adapting accordingly. This is known as *adaptive management*. It is widely used in environmental engineering and IT, and it ought to be used more and more in health care. Adaptive project management offers learning based on actual project performance, through testing. It requires that we admit flaws and failings, and that we modify the project to incorporate what we have learned. As we will see in the following chapter, it also requires the ability to let go of ineffective and underperforming projects rather than investing more money and more time in the hope of reviving them. The fact that an organization has already put a lot of money into an initiative—the "sunk costs" theory—is never a good reason for maintaining a failing or a failed project.

Milestones, stage gates, and key performance indicators can play a role in mitigating risk, too; if you aren't reaching your targets along the way, you know that something is going wrong. We will discuss these in chapter 3 as well.

SUMMARY

- Every initiative can be judged by two essential criteria: Is it the right thing to be doing? And is the change team going about it in the right way?

- Traditional measures of success—scope, cost, and time—are insufficient in health care. Change events must also "stay live," be fit for use, and minimize risk.

- Risk analysis is especially critical. Planners need to determine how to mitigate risk, avoid it, transfer it, or accept it.

NOTES

1. Ivars Avots, "Why Does Project Management Fail?" *California Management Review* 12, no. 1 (Fall 1969): 77.
2. Sandra G. Boodman, "The Pain of Wrong-Site Surgery," *Washington Post*, June 20, 2011.
3. David A. Shore, Christina Lively, and Towers Watson, *The Hospital Industry in Transition: Building Capability to Successfully Drive Change* (San Francisco: Towers Watson, 2011), http://www.towerswatson.com/DownloadMedia.aspx?media=%7BCF62E9 B2-2195-4DDC-BE75-FA9730B8282A%D.
4. For a more detailed discussion of these concepts, see Erik W. Gray and Clifford F. Larson, *Project Management: The Managerial Process* (New York: McGraw-Hill, 2008).

3

Planning: Seeds of Success and Failure

Recent research into Alzheimer's disease has uncovered a sad truth: the illness has an extended preclinical stage that may last as long as ten years. During this phase the patient has no symptoms, but recognizable changes in the brain are already occurring. Autopsy reports reveal that a high percentage of people with undetected early-onset Alzheimer's were often mistakenly diagnosed with other forms of dementia. Forty-seven percent were still incorrectly diagnosed at the time of death. Moreover, of people with atypical symptoms and no memory problems, 53 percent were incorrectly diagnosed.[1] Today, doctors can probe the neurons of potential Alzheimer's patients before they show symptoms. In theory, neuroimaging can be used to identify neurological changes and predict a person's risk of developing the disease. New clinical guidelines and recommendations therefore focus on early detection, before the onset of dementia that is characteristic of Alzheimer's. This enables patients to receive medication that could help slow the progress of the disease.

Alzheimer's is hardly unique in this regard. Thanks to modern diagnostic technologies, the preclinical stages of many illnesses are becoming familiar to physicians and other clinicians. As a result, health care practitioners are learning that they can intervene earlier, often with better results than in the past. The preclinical stage, after all, contains the seeds of later systemic clinical failures. If those seeds can be eradicated or controlled early on, the chances of a positive outcome are that much greater.

This book is about the beginning of a health care project. The beginning is like the preclinical stage of an initiative. What happens during this time is critical. Depending on how you approach it, it may contain the seeds of failure or the seeds of success. To change the metaphor for a moment, it is like the takeoff phase of an airplane flight. A lot has to happen during this phase, and it all has to go right. If it does not go right, the flight will not succeed. With planning, the objective is both to identify potential risks in advance and to mitigate risks as early as possible when they do occur.

Parts 2 and 3 of the book will examine the two key tasks for this phase, selecting the right projects and choosing the right people. This chapter focuses on something that must precede any project or people selection: planning.

A TIME FOR PLANNING

Planning is a time-honored desideratum. Alexander Graham Bell, echoing Confucius, said, "Before anything else, preparation is the key to success." Winston Churchill declared, "He who fails to plan is planning to fail." Yogi Berra put it only a little differently: "If you don't know where you're going," he said, "you might not get there." The syntax is characteristically labored but the meaning is clear.

The trouble is, we human beings often do not plan effectively. (Perhaps that is why so many sages felt compelled to pronounce upon the importance of planning.) We hope for the best. We learn as we go. We wing it. The result with change initiatives, typically, is scope creep, delays, cost overruns, unforeseen challenges, and ultimately a loss of faith in the whole enterprise.

Health care organizations seem to be particularly bad at planning. Many do little planning except for with their largest and most complex projects, such as a new building. They are apt to launch an initiative to define a new operating room procedure or intake process purely on the basis of an idea rather than a plan. Even some big projects suffer from poor planning. Look, for example, at what has happened so far—up to early 2014—with the attempt to create accountable care organizations (ACOs), the new medical model encouraged by the Patient Protection and Affordable Care Act, America's 2010 health care reform law. The start-up and first-year costs of the nation's fledgling ACOs have turned out to be between six and fourteen times higher than the original estimates from the Department of Health and Human Services. Even allowing for a little self-interest—the figures are from a survey conducted by the American Hospital Association—that is rather a large gap.[2]

As one wit put it, projects typically begin with a lot of pondering, which then proceeds to procrastination and ends up in panic. Nor do health care leaders usually track performance in relation to the original plan. (Difficult to do if there's no plan to start with!) Most executives do not even know how many projects are under way in their organization, let alone where they are in the project life cycle or how they are performing.

Why is planning hard? Several factors are at work. Everyone feels an incentive to act, to do things. No one's job description includes "*Think.*" Few hospitals and health care systems have a project management methodology; rather, they follow Nike's slogan and "just do it." Leaders tend to be impatient, wanting things to happen quickly. Yet the seeds of failure for new initiatives take root early in the life cycle of a project. Without a plan, no one may even recognize that those seeds are germinating.

Good planning pays off many times over. It helps put projects on the right track—and keep them there—in at least five ways:

- **A plan is a gauge for measuring progress.** Project teams often do not report their findings and results until the end of the initiative. It makes more sense, however, to establish milestones and require reporting along the way, with specific deliverables at each of the various tollgates tied to funding. If the project is on track, it qualifies for additional funding and can continue. If not, it can be modified or terminated. This pay-to-play approach stands in stark contrast to today's typical process, whereby health care systems fund entire projects up front at the time of project approval.

- **A plan shifts the "worry curve."** As I noted in chapter 2, every project is an experiment; every project entails risk. Nobody knows the outcome, and the estimates are likely to be off base. But the absence of certainty should not lead to the conclusion that planning is irrelevant. Good planning reduces risk and makes it more likely that the outcome will turn out as desired. It enables project team members to map out in advance what they want to have happen. It helps teams understand that it is acceptable not to know everything. It gives them a license to discover what they need to know and conduct a "rethink" when necessary. No student pilot would accept an assignment to taxi down the runway at takeoff speed without a great deal of advance preparation.

- **A plan saves money.** When you build a house, the cheapest dollar is always the design dollar. The design stage is when you can reconsider your ideas, redraw the design, even start over, all at relatively minimal cost. In change initiatives, the cheapest dollar is the planning dollar. An extended planning stage allows you to estimate your efforts forward into the future, assessing the likelihood of various scenarios and revising your plans accordingly. If you begin to implement a plan and then must change it, the change is always more cumbersome and costly than it would have been at an earlier stage.

- **A plan allows for strategic sequencing.** Projects unfold in phases. Any IT project, for instance, involves extensive planning, then coding, testing, debugging, further testing and debugging, and finally "going live." Clinical projects may be piloted in a small unit, then rolled out to an entire organization. A good plan spells out the sequence of phases so that the project team can focus on what needs to be done now rather than on what should be done at a later stage.

- **A plan gives team members the opportunity to propose pulling the plug.** The signs of project failure are often first visible to team members themselves. People stop coming to meetings. Executives lose interest. There are cost surprises, changes in the environment or competitive landscape, or changes in the leadership and direction of the organization. There are technological, regulatory, or ethical issues raised by the project—or maybe the project is so far off plan that it is hard to imagine that it will ever succeed. The health care industry, however, is notorious for never pulling the plug on projects. People miss or suppress these warning signs because they want to report good news, or because they fear repercussions. Team members must recognize that proposing to pull the plug on a failing project will be viewed as good and even heroic, not as a career-ending decision.

A project in many ways is a grand learning experience. The first mile is no exception. Though the project is only in the planning stages, team members should be learning every day. They try out ideas among themselves. They ask for feedback on their plans from coworkers and other stakeholders. If they go about things right, they will be far wiser at the end of the planning phase than they were at the beginning.

LEARNING FROM FAILURE

Many people in health care are familiar with the phrase *amenable mortality*. It is a statistic measuring deaths that are potentially preventable with timely and effective health care. Amenable mortality—which includes deaths in patients only up to age seventy-five—is a significant proportion of total mortality in every country. The United States rates poorly on this measure; in a 2002–2003 study of Organisation for Economic Co-operation and Development countries, it came in dead last, with a rate of 110 preventable deaths per 100,000. There was more than a twofold variation across the states, from a low of 63.9 in Minnesota to a high of 158.3 in the District of Columbia.[3]

In projects, as in medicine, people often plan for success. They map out what is supposed to happen and ignore the possibility that something else entirely might happen. The project dies—even though its troubles might have been foreseen, or discovered along the way. It suffers from amenable mortality. The single most important antidote to amenable mortality in projects is to learn from experience. Oddly, that seems to be particularly difficult for many health care organizations to do. How difficult? Consider this homely example. In the past couple of decades, many hospitals around the country launched a significant project: they changed their name from "hospital" to "medical center." The word *hospital* was old fashioned, administrators felt. The words *medical center* conjured up a twenty-first-century organization with leading-edge technology. Every one of these changes was a significant undertaking and undoubtedly cost a substantial amount of money.

There was just one problem: the public preferred the word *hospital.* In a 2002 poll, a plurality of respondents said that "hospitals" rather than "medical centers" offered a wider range of services, provided better-quality care, and used the most advanced procedures.[4] Nevertheless, the trend toward renaming continued. In 2011 the same pollsters repeated the poll—and found much the same results. Asked, "Which has a wider range of services?" for example, 61 percent of respondents said "hospitals," compared to 31 percent for "medical centers." In 2002 the numbers were 56 percent and 35 percent.[5] Hospitals continued to change their names even after polling evidence confirmed twice in a decade that this was unwise.

In projects and initiatives, we have to learn from failure at an organizational level. We have to do better the second time—and the third and the fourth time—than we did the first time. The army knows this, which is why it regularly conducts what it calls an after-action review. Football teams know it as well; they look at videos of the previous game and try to codify what they have learned. Yet health care organizations and project teams are notorious for not learning from failure. They do not compile the lessons learned, or they do so in a perfunctory manner. They do not document what they have learned, or share it with others. At best, they capture lessons learned at the end of a project rather than all along the way, with the result that the "lessons" all have to do with what happened at the project's close. To be sure, health care isn't unique in this respect. According to one study, only 12 percent of senior executives believe that their organization does a good job of sharing knowledge.[6]

Of all the opportunities for increasing the success rate of projects, this may be the most profound. Organizations that excel at improvement projects have processes in place to capture lessons learned at every phase. They conduct regular reviews of a project's progress, both after each milestone and whenever they learn something that will contribute to improved performance. The reviewers undertake such tasks as determining the continuing feasibility of the project, checking to be sure all necessary activities have been completed before presenting a solution to a problem, and tracking deviations and variances from the plan. This kind of learning takes place at the team level as well. As the project proceeds, the team notes and records what is working and what is not working, and takes effective countermeasures to address the latter. If the project fails completely, team members conduct a detailed postmortem to see what went wrong, so that they can identify and fix critical barriers to the success of the next project. Reviewing lessons learned from past projects is all part of effective planning.

Successful organizations also make sure that lessons are not just learned but also *leveraged* by creating searchable databases of lessons from past projects, including relevant tools, techniques, and advice. Project teams routinely search this database whenever a new initiative begins. The goal is to reduce the amenable mortality rate of projects.

It is hard to overestimate the value of this kind of learning. But seasoned leaders know its importance. In the early years of IBM—it was then called International Business Machines—company president Thomas J. Watson called an executive into his office. The executive had made a dramatic error in judgment that cost the company $30,000, which in those days was a large sum even for IBM. The executive was pretty sure he would be fired.

Watson walked the executive through his mistake, asking what had led to the error and helping him see how it could have been avoided. The executive found this to be slow torture and asked his chief why he didn't just get it over with and fire him.

"Fire you?" Watson asked in disbelief. "Why would we fire you when we have just spent $30,000 educating you!"

Like Watson, a good project team surfaces its mistakes and mis-judgments, even in the planning phase. It reviews them, asks why they happened, and makes better plans for the future. In this way, project success begins well before implementation even commences. It begins during the takeoff phase, before anything is in the air.

• • •

I began this chapter with a medical analogy, and I want to end with one as well. The Nuka System of Care is the "name given to the whole health care system created, managed, and owned by Alaska Native people to achieve physical, mental, emotional, and spiritual wellness."[7] It addresses the needs of a community with a high incidence of disease, and it has achieved remarkable results on virtually every metric that gauges quality of life.

The system is based on a premise known as "five-year gestation." If you can keep a baby in good health for its first five years, you have helped it on the road to good health for the next seventy. This premise has much support in the medical literature. Studies have found that adverse childhood experiences (such as physical or emotional abuse or family dysfunction) bear a strong relationship to later health and well-being.[8] The Nuka system focuses on the period before conception, on pregnancy, on the birth-to-two-months phase, and on two months to five years. The idea is to have a beneficial long-range impact by concentrating efforts on the early years.

As with children, so with projects: start them right.

SUMMARY

- Many health care organizations don't take planning seriously. Yet good planning pays for itself many times over.

- Planning is both a gauge for measuring progress and a money saver. It allows teams to shift the "worry curve," sequence events appropriately, and propose pulling the plug when necessary.

- In particular, spotlighting failure enables a team to capture lessons learned when things don't go as expected.

NOTES

1. Michael Balasa et al., "Clinical Features and APOE Genotype of Pathologically Proven Early-Onset Alzheimer Disease," *Neurology* 76 (May 2011): 1720–1725; Mason A. Israel et al., "Probing Sporadic and Familial Alzheimer's Disease Using Induced Pluripotent Stem Cells," *Nature* 482, no. 7384 (January 2012): 216–220. See also Reisa A. Sperling et al., "Toward Defining the Preclinical Stages of Alzheimer's Disease: Recommendations from the National Institute on Aging and the Alzheimer's Association Workgroup," *Journal of the Alzheimer's Association* 7, no. 3 (May 2011): 280–292.

2. American Hospital Association, "New Study Finds the Start Up Costs of Establishing an ACO to Be Significant. CMS Underestimates the Investment Needed to Create an ACO," news release, May 13, 2011, http://www.aha.org/advocacy-issues/clininteg /casestudies.shtml.

3. Stephen C. Schoenbaum et al., "Mortality Amenable to Health Care in the United States: The Roles of Demographics and Health System Performance," *Journal of Public Health Policy* 32 (2011): 407–429.

4. "A Hospital by Any Other Name Doesn't Seem So Cutting-Edge," *Modern Healthcare* 32, no. 14 (April 2002): 36.

5. See http://www.baumanresearch.com/hospitalsurvey.

6. See, for example, Gabriel Szulanski and Sidney Winter, "Getting It Right the Second Time," *Harvard Business Review* 80, no. 1 (January 2002): 62–69.

7. See http://www.scf.cc/nuka/index.ak.

8. See this pathbreaking study: Vincent J. Felitti et al., "The Relationship of Adult Health Status to Childhood Abuse and Household Dysfunction," *American Journal of Preventive Medicine* 14, no. 4 (May 1998): 245–258, http://www.ncbi.nim.nih .gov/pubmed/9635069.

PART 2

Select the Right Projects

INTRODUCTION: THE CROWDED RUNWAY

Physicians and other clinicians often do too much. They prescribe antibiotics for sinus infections and proton-pump inhibitors for heartburn. They give stress tests to healthy people and cancer tests to dialysis patients. They order X-rays for lower-back pain and brain scans for fainting. These are just a few of the procedures that patients should question, according to a coalition of specialty societies representing some 375,000 U.S. physicians.[1] Sometimes the treatment or test is appropriate. Even so, it is often unnecessary as defined in standard medical practice, or overly aggressive, and the procedure becomes part of the estimated 30 percent of health care spending that is wasted.[2]

Health care organizations are like the clinicians they support: they, too, try to do too much. They have too many initiatives under way, and they launch more all the time. Talk to anyone who works for a health care organization, and you are likely to hear the same refrains: "We're swamped." "We're buried." "We have more projects than we can possibly handle." Projects are stacked up like airplanes on a runway before a thunderstorm, and the people who are supposed to be implementing those initiatives are overwhelmed.

Why so many projects? Let me count the reasons.

Reason one: ideas for change initiatives come from all over. Some are imposed from the outside by new regulations or requirements. Some come bubbling up from physicians and other clinicians, and from departments such as IT and human resources. Many managers and executives have their pet projects. Most people who work in health care have experienced what might be termed *in-flight magazine syndrome*. A leader returns from a trip having attended a conference or—worse—having read a business magazine on the plane back. Suddenly he or she has half a dozen ideas for new projects and would like to see them implemented right away. Improvements in health care management and clinical patient management, not to mention an overall environment of innovative processes in business, leave most hospitals scrambling to keep up. And keeping up with clinical and business improvements means implementing more change initiatives in the organization.

Reason two: health care organizations have a hard time saying no to project ideas. That may be because so few organizations have a systematic approach, like that provided by this book, to selecting and managing projects. Instead, the process unfolds something like this. Somebody gets an idea and brings it to a few other people. The other people are encouraging, and the originator develops it further. Finally he or she takes the idea to an executive, maybe with a small group coming along in support. The executive agrees to the project, usually thinking, *Well, what harm can it do? It may even work, and we will be better off. Besides, those people seemed very enthusiastic. I hate to be the bad guy.*

Reason three: people fall in love with their projects. Once people launch a project, they desperately want it to succeed. They may even feel that their professional reputation is at stake. I think of this particular disease as "projectitis," and I find in my work that it infects a lot of people. When you are in love with something, you will fight tooth and nail to keep it. You will greet all who presume to question it with a barrage of renewed determination and enthusiasm, hoping to quell their criticisms. (P.S. It usually works. The critics go away, and the project limps on.)

Reason four: change initiatives are *hard*. They typically require people to change their behaviors or their accustomed ways of doing things. That provokes a lot of opposition from the people affected. The pushback leads to requests to modify or delay the project, to gather more data, or to consider different approaches. Those requests, in turn, mean that most projects take far longer than planned and technically remain active even if progress is slow or stalled.

Reason five, which in some ways is the most basic of all: too many projects never die. You can think of them, using the imagery that has become popular among teenagers, as zombies. Zombie projects are the living dead of health care organizations. Such projects have never been formally terminated, so they are still on the books. The groups responsible for them may hold occasional meetings, but nothing much happens. The organization has no mechanism for reviewing, monitoring, or terminating initiatives, and so each one lives on until it finally accomplishes its objectives or—more commonly—fades slowly into obscurity.

The conventional approach to initiatives among health care organizations can be described as "spray and pray." That is a harsh judgment, but there is considerable truth to it. There is no central nervous system that guides an organization in its choices, no rational or systematic method of choosing which initiatives to invest in and which not. Organizations thus waste resources on projects that don't fit with their mission. They waste resources on projects that are well intentioned but poorly executed, and so don't accomplish much. They raise people's expectations that something good might actually happen from all these projects; indeed, some initiatives are launched with a great deal of fanfare. But then nothing changes, and employees begin to roll their eyes whenever the next one appears. Many organizations suffer from the maladies of workplace demoralization and cynicism; health care organizations are no exception.

So this part of the book is about creating a mechanism for selecting projects, and about the process for doing so. In the following chapters we will examine how a health care organization can develop and identify the right initiatives, and how it can choose and prioritize those initiatives. We will also look closely at how it can monitor the initiatives, supporting or terminating them when it is appropriate to do so. Our guiding principle is from Goethe: "Things that matter most must never be at the mercy of things that matter least." Finally, medicine has comparative effectiveness research, which aims to distinguish treatments and tests that work from those that do not. Health care organizations need something similar when it comes to projects: they need to know what is likely to work and what is already working, and they need to know what is superfluous or simply wasteful. Then they need to apply that knowledge by selecting and supporting and maintaining only the *right* projects—the ones that matter most.

The late Steve Jobs is widely remembered and respected for his leading role in creating a wildly successful company, Apple. What we often forget is how fiercely Jobs had to struggle, and how much he had to learn, on the path to success. In 1983, when Jobs was only twenty-eight, he recruited John Sculley away from PepsiCo to become CEO of Apple, with the understanding that the two of them would run the company together. The partnership did not work out, and two years later Jobs was eased out of the company he cofounded by Sculley and the board of directors. When Jobs returned to Apple in 1997, he found a company in disarray—mostly because it was trying to do too much. "The company was churning out multiple versions of each product because of bureaucratic momentum and to satisfy the whims of retailers," wrote Walter Isaacson in his biography of Jobs. "Apple had a dozen versions of the Macintosh, each with a different confusing number, ranging from 1400 to 9600. 'I had people explaining this to me for three weeks,' Jobs said. 'I couldn't figure it out.' He finally began asking simple questions, like 'Which ones do I tell my friends to buy?'"

Soon Jobs began cutting product lines, individual models, and variations. He ended Apple's foray into the printer business. He killed troubled products, such as the Newton, an early personal digital device. All told, he ended up eliminating more than 70 percent of the products and models Apple had been selling or developing. At one product strategy session, he famously listened to people debating this or that version of an Apple computer and then yelled, "Stop!" Going to a whiteboard, he told the group, "Here's what we need." He drew a two-by-two matrix on the board, with the columns labeled "Consumer" and "Pro" and the rows labeled "Desktop" and "Portable." The group's job, he told them, "was to make four great products, one for each quadrant."[3]

That would become one of Apple's hallmarks under Jobs: a relentless focus on just a handful of product families, not too many varieties or variations, no ventures into businesses away from Apple's—sorry—core. "I'm actually as proud of what we don't do as of what we do do," he said, meaning that you can't do great things unless you quit wasting your resources in areas where you will never be great. Following that philosophy, Jobs created what ultimately became one of the world's most valuable companies.

Health care companies cannot follow Jobs's model exactly. They cannot say, "We don't do a good job at insurance collection, so we will just eliminate it." But they can observe the spirit of Jobs's actions, and never let the things that matter least get in the way of the things that matter most. In particular, they can focus their change efforts on the few areas that they deem most important. The information imparted in the chapters that follow could help them decide—and be proud of—what they should not do as well as what they should do.

SUMMARY

- Health care organizations typically have far too many projects under way at once. It's a "spray-and-pray" approach, without any central strategy or guidance.

- Most need a mechanism for selecting the right projects—and for deselecting everything else. As at Apple, what you *don't* do can be as important as what you do.

NOTES

1. See American Board of Internal Medicine Foundation, Choosing Wisely, http://choosingwisely.org/.
2. See, for example, David Lawrence, "Bridging the Quality Chasm," in *Building a Better Delivery System: A New Engineering/Health Care Partnership*, ed. Proctor P. Reid et al. (Washington, DC: National Academies Press, 2005), http://www.nap.edu/openbook.php?record_id=11378&page=R1.
3. Walter Isaacson, *Steve Jobs* (New York: Simon & Schuster, 2011), 337.

4

Identifying and Creating the Right Initiatives

In the not-too-distant past, the job of big-city police officers on a beat was mostly to ride around in a car keeping an eye on things and waiting for a call. The policing system was essentially passive: it rarely swung into action until a crime was committed and someone called for help.

Today, policing in most U.S. cities, particularly New York, is far more proactive. Computer-driven statistics show exactly what happened during the last week or month in each district or precinct. Precinct commanders are held accountable for reducing crime in the areas for which they are responsible. Among the tactics used is so-called hot-spot policing. "The great majority of crimes tend to occur in the same places," explained the late social scientist James Q. Wilson. "Put active police resources in those areas instead of telling officers to drive around waiting for 911 calls, and you can bring down crime."[1] The change in police tactics is generally thought to be one of the factors contributing to the notable decline in crime rates in most parts of the United States during the 1990s and 2000s.

Health care, too, has undergone a shift—or, more accurately, is in the midst of one. The earlier model was passive, much like the police's approach. Physicians and other clinicians waited until people showed up at their offices. Hospitals and medical centers waited until patients requested admission or turned up in the emergency room. Insurance companies and other payers waited until a member filed a claim. Like the police, the system would swing into action once a relevant event occurred.

Though that model still dominates today, expectations and practices are shifting rapidly in the direction of a more active approach to health care. All three of these stakeholder groups, and many others, do their best to encourage good health habits and preventive care. Gradually, and with the encouragement of the health care reform law of 2010 in the United States, health care provider organizations are beginning to assume accountability for entire episodes of care, for successful outcomes, and for patients' overall well-being. Health care is shifting from *volume* to *value*. Increasingly, the measure of success is no longer how many patients you treat but how well you care for them and whether or not you improve their health.

This shift needs to be reflected in organizations' approaches to change initiatives. Rather than passively waiting for ideas to come along and then trying them out to see whether they work, health care organizations need to be identifying, developing, and selecting the ideas that will make a difference. They need to be *proactive*, both in clarifying their goals and in pursuing the proposals that will bring them closer to those objectives. They need to view change initiatives as part of the strategic planning that will get them *from* where they are now *to* where they want to be. If an initiative doesn't help on that journey, it has no place in the organization. The most important question, in short, is no longer "How can we do it faster?" or "How can we do it cheaper?" or even "How can we do it better?" The most important question is, "Why do we do it at all?"

CHANGE INITIATIVES AS STRATEGIC PLANNING

In the previous paragraph I referred to a health care organization's "goals." That was just convenient shorthand, which we can now dispense with. Before a health care organization can have goals, it must have a mission, a vision, and values. In my presentations I usually abbreviate these terms as MV^2. Many people remark that they find this a useful device for remembering these three key concepts.[2]

An organization's *mission* is its purpose, a description of why it exists. Johnson & Johnson says, "The fundamental objective of Johnson & Johnson is to provide scientifically sound, high quality products and services to help heal, cure disease and improve the quality of life." Pfizer says, "We dedicate ourselves to humanity's quest for longer, healthier, happier lives through innovation in pharmaceutical, consumer, and animal health products." Children's Hospitals and Clinics, in Minneapolis–St. Paul, says this:

> Children's Hospitals and Clinics champions the special health needs of children and their families. We are committed to improving children's health by providing high-quality, family-centered pediatric services. We advance these efforts through research and education.

These missions are broadly stated, to be sure. A smaller organization might have a more limited mission. Whatever the scope, the fundamental idea of a mission is simplicity itself: this is our raison d'être. This is why we get up in the morning. If the people who work in your organization do not know what its mission is, how can you expect them to understand which change initiatives matter and which do not?

An organization's *vision*, in contrast, describes where it is headed, what it wants to become. Missions are timeless, but visions are very much time bound: "This is where we want to be in five years," or "This is where we want to be in ten years." Words like *leading* or *preeminent* often appear in vision statements, because organizations often aspire to be the best. A vision brings a sense of movement, of progress, to an organization: "We are headed in this direction, and we are on the way." Conversely, an organization without an explicit vision is like a plane with no destination, aimlessly flying around. And what can that ever lead to? "If you don't know where you're going," said Yogi Berra, "you might not get there."

An organization's *values*, finally, define how it wants employees to act and not act as they pursue the vision. Perhaps the organization values integrity or teamwork. Perhaps its emphasis is on quality or on innovation. A statement of just a few central values helps remind everyone what the expectations are. They should pursue the vision, but only within the framework established by the values.

MV^2 sets the context for strategic planning, and you cannot do strategic planning without MV^2. Strategic planning determines how the organization will implement its mission. It determines how and when and at what cost it will realize its vision.

What Strategic Planning Is

Health care is essentially a system designed to move people from one state of affairs to a better one—from sickness to health, from a debilitating condition to a salubrious one. It is all about moving *from* one point *to* another point. The same can be said of strategic planning. It answers the overarching question: "How do we get from where we are now to where we want to be?" Any number of questions can be subsumed in that broad interrogative. "What new services should we deliver? Do we need to expand? Which facilities or processes need to be fixed or replaced? How can we improve the quality of our care?" These are questions that health care administrators and executives ask themselves all the time, of course, but my point is that they can be answered effectively only within the context of a strategic plan.

A good strategic plan has at least three characteristics.

First, it lays out measurable objectives. These are the goals—often stretch goals, ambitious but still possible—that will advance progress toward the organization's vision. The goals might include measures of care quality, efficiency, and cost. They might include external metrics, such as improvement in regard to an organization's reputation, market share, or standing in the community, or perhaps its success in raising capital. The objectives naturally differ from year to year, depending on the organization's situation. One year's goals might include, "Expand capacity by 20 percent through acquisition." The following year's goals might include, "Integrate the facilities we acquired through standardized systems and procedures."

Second, the strategic plan maps out *how* each objective will be accomplished. Not in the details—this is a strategic plan, not an action plan—but in general. The objectives, in other words, are not simply a wish list of pie-in-the-sky, nice-to-have ends; they are real-world goals, and they are tied to an understanding of how the organization will pursue them. A nonprofit medical center, for example, cannot simply state a goal of raising an additional $3 million in philanthropic contributions. The plan has to include a broad outline of which groups of individuals or philanthropies the organization will target and how it will position its requests. That is why the plan is called *strategic*.

Third, the plan links its objectives and methods to a budget.

This last bears an additional word of explanation. Every organization has a budget, and virtually every organization engages in an annual budgeting process. The process often involves negotiations between administrators or finance staff and the heads of individual departments and divisions. Most commonly, the budget for next year is pegged to the budget for this year, and the organization is looking for a small increase or decrease. This kind of incremental budgeting—all too common in health care, as in other industries—is not strategic planning. It assumes that all we want to do is pretty much what we did before. There is no sense of movement, of progress toward a goal, of accomplishment. And there are no deliberate choices about where the organization should spend its money or to what it should devote its time.

That is why a true strategic plan is intimately linked to a budget and a budget is intimately linked to a strategic plan. The plan comes first. But it is never divorced from fiscal realities, and it may need to be modified in light of budgetary restrictions. An organization with a strategic plan thus knows not only where it is going—from here to there—but also how much the trip will cost. Ensuring affordability is an essential part of the plan. The plan connects goals to available resources.

Organizations have a variety of methods for creating strategic plans. They may gather a team of senior executives to go off-site and map out priorities. They may request a plan (as well as a budget) from each unit head, and then integrate them. Often, the chief executive may take the lead; board members may or may not be involved. This is not a book about strategic planning, so I will not go into detail. The only idea I want to leave you with is that strategic planning is an essential part of running an organization, an indispensable factor in success. It is crucial that all the relevant stakeholders buy into and feel inspired by the strategic plan. If you do not have a well-thought-out, broadly accepted strategic plan, you will not know how to allocate your resources. And that, of course, means that you will be unable to select the right change initiatives.

Strategic Planning and Initiatives

Change initiatives or projects are the *method* by which an organization pursues its strategic plan and ultimately realizes its vision. Clinical interventions move patients from one state to a better one. Initiatives move organizations from one state to a better one. The strategic plan provides the framework into which the initiatives must fit.

That said, a strategic plan must also be flexible enough to accommodate the projects that are considered "must-do's." Consider the recent push for health care organizations of all sorts to create electronic health records (EHRs). Many physician practices, hospitals, and other organizations have been dragging their feet in computerizing patient records, but even the laggards are coming to see that they can no longer avoid creating EHRs. In the United States, a combination of regulations and incentives is likely to tip the balance and make EHRs far more common than they are at this writing. By now, in fact, any organization that does not have EHRs is likely to include them as part of a future strategic plan.

However, a strategic plan should never be simply a response to outside requirements; it should shape and frame those requirements, and spell out why, how, and toward what end the organization will respond to them. For example, computerizing patient records may provide a health care organization with an opportunity to improve patient care. The task may be part of becoming an accountable care organization. It may enable the organization to gain an advantage over the competition by making its records faster,

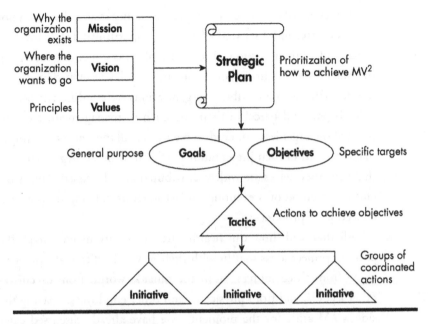

Figure 4.1   Strategic Planning and Initiatives

better, and more user friendly. These are all objectives that could be part of a strategic plan, and the project of computerizing records would fit nicely into it.

To recap, MV^2 and the strategic plan that derives from it should always guide project planning and implementation (figure 4.1). Now let us look more closely at where projects come from. We will then be well positioned to consider in chapter 5 how to select, prioritize, and monitor them.

WHERE GOOD PROJECT IDEAS ORIGINATE

Health care organizations already have plenty of projects, as we have seen. The difficulty is that those projects often do not come from the right sources, and they do not always fit with an organization's MV^2. How can that be changed?

The essential antidote, if you are not doing it already, is to publicize, communicate, and discuss MV^2 at every opportunity. Too many organizations think of their mission, vision, and values as something for a plaque on the wall of the boardroom, or as something to be developed by the marketing department. Vital, vibrant organizations have a different perspective. MV^2 is part and parcel of their approach to management, a critical element of the organization. Leaders mention it all the time at meetings. They make it a part of their presentations. MV^2 informs strategic planning, and the plans themselves are widely distributed and discussed. This is the *only* effective method of preventing project ideas from being simply a random collection of proposals.

All that said, how can health care organizations encourage the creation of project ideas that fit with their MV^2? Traditionally, projects have come from three sources: from the outside world, from executives and other leaders, and from physicians and other employees. Leaving the outside world aside for the moment—we have already discussed externally inspired projects—we can think of projects as either top down or bottom up. Top-down projects are usually the creation of a small group of managers or executives and are wished on those below them. (This category includes the pet projects mentioned earlier.) Bottom-up projects are the creation of employees and only later get the imprimatur of management. I propose a different way of thinking of project creation, one that involves dialogue between leaders and the rank and file.

- **Listening sessions**. What would happen, for example, if unit leaders and other administrators regularly conducted listening sessions? Imagine that they attended unit meetings with their ears open and their mouths mostly shut. They would begin to get a sense of the pain points, the daily frustrations, the obstacles that prevent people in the unit from doing a better job, or from fulfilling their part of the organization's vision. Several weeks' worth of input from this source would no doubt lead to a number of good project ideas, each of them informed by MV^2. Is this top down or bottom up? It is really neither one. The whole process is based on dialogue.

- **Gemba walks**. *Gemba* in Japanese refers to the real place, the place where things happen, the place where the work is done. A *gemba walk* is simply a walk through a portion of the workplace with specific objectives and questions in mind.[3] How do people create value? Where are they wasting time or resources? What would need to happen to increase value creation and decrease waste? A good gemba walk has a specific theme and focuses on a particular set of interactions. The leader performing the walk does not look for everything; he or she looks for certain critical processes and ways of doing things. But it is essential to look at everything that falls within that purview. In the lab, for instance, how are blood samples taken, labeled, and stored? How are patients scheduled and processed? What is the patient's experience in visiting the lab? What is the communication between receptionist and technician? Informed observation is likely to reveal many activities that do not necessarily serve a patient's or the organization's best interests.

- **A culture of innovation**. Innovation specialists in other industries regularly emphasize the importance of a *culture* of innovation. Such companies as Procter & Gamble and Apple go to great lengths to make innovation a part of what people think about every day. In health care, most innovation occurs through change initiatives or projects, and the same rule applies. You want to create an environment in which large numbers of people are thinking about how to make things better, and about how they might develop a project to do so. Projects should never be the responsibility of a small group of individuals, however that group might be defined. Successful innovators always tap the ideas of as many people as possible.

DEVELOPING PROJECT CONCEPTS

Now let us imagine that someone—I call that person the concept initiator—has come up with an idea. How does he or she develop and evaluate it?

This is the *concept exploration phase* of projects, and it is essential to a good launch. It is like an initial screen. If a project never makes it out of this phase, the organization has been spared the time and expense necessary to review a poorly conceived project. If it does make it out, the odds that the project will be successful are far higher than they otherwise would be. The concept initiator discusses the idea with relevant individuals, collecting feedback. He or she may want to conduct a precedence study, as architects and engineers often do. Particularly in health care, it is likely that someone, somewhere, has tried something similar, with results either positive or negative. Reviewing the results of somebody else's experiment is a particularly inexpensive way of assessing the potential of a project idea.

The initiator must then ask him- or herself a series of questions. The questions are not definitive; rather, they create an early stage gate to help determine whether the idea is worth pursuing. Among them might be the following:

- What is the project's goal? Why is this goal important?
- What is the current process, and what do we propose to replace it with? Why is our replacement better?
- Who will be affected by this change event?
- How will these stakeholders be affected?
- How can we get buy-in from essential groups?
- How will success be measured and tracked?

If the idea "passes" these initial critical questions, it is time for a more rigorous analysis that will locate the proposed idea in the context of the organization's needs. Answering questions such as the following requires deeper analysis. They put the idea to a more strenuous test.

- **How does this idea align with the organization's strategic needs?** A key consideration should be assessment of a project's desired outcomes in the context of the organization's mission, vision, values, and strategic plan. To which strategy in particular does this initiative contribute? What clinical or business problem does it solve?

- **What is the risk involved?** The trajectory of every change initiative is unpredictable, and the outcome is uncertain. The project may not work as designed. It may work as designed but have unintended and unexpected consequences. It may cost more—sometimes far more—than planned. All these risks have to be factored into a proposal. So, too, does the risk of not undertaking the proposal at all. Health care, like life, involves sins of omission as well as sins of commission.

- **What are the likely costs compared to the probable benefits?** The initiator needs to examine both direct and indirect costs in relation to estimated benefits. Costs, of course, include both financial outlays and time spent on the project. In most cases the project should show a positive return on investment.

- **In what ways would the project's desired outcomes benefit end users and other stakeholders?** The earlier screen helps the initiator determine some of the benefits. But any health care organization is a complex system, with multiple objectives and a variety of stakeholders. A project with clear benefits for the pharmacy department may make life more difficult for physicians. Every stakeholder's interests need to be taken into account.

- **Does this project fit with our organization's culture?** This question is essential to ask, but the answer can cut both ways. A project that fits well with the culture naturally will have an easier time of it. Sometimes, however, the very purpose of an initiative is to begin—or contribute to—changing the culture. In that case a "no" answer is not necessarily a deal breaker. In any case, the impact of culture on the project should be considered.

- **What is the timeline—and how will we know whether we are succeeding?** This is a restatement of the "measuring success" question asked early on, but it involves an all-important addition: the notion of a timeline, and of measuring points along the way.

Tracking an initiative involves knowing whether it is on course as it proceeds, not just evaluating it at the end. Any good proposal requires metrics and milestones.

The Plan of Concept

Organizations that have a formal system for initiating and managing projects typically require a "proof of concept" document prior to approval, and then prepare a project charter once the idea has been approved. What we are discussing now is something needed at an earlier stage in the process. I call it a *plan* of concept, and it is far less detailed than either of the other two documents. At this stage a health care organization is not necessarily looking for detailed, well-supported answers to every question about the proposed project. It is—or it should be—looking for evidence that the concept initiator has given some thought to these issues, and that he or she has reasonable answers at hand. The initiator should be able to give a persuasive presentation or write-up explaining in broad strokes why the proposed idea is a good use of the organization's resources; what the value proposition of the idea is; why it is likely to be more effective than current practices; how it fits with the strategic plan; and how it serves the needs of customers and other stakeholders. The initiator should know in rough terms how the project will evolve, who will be involved in it, how much it will cost, and how its progress can be assessed.

In some cases the plan of concept will explicitly describe an experiment. Experiments differ from other projects. Instead of proposing to move the organization from point A to point B, they propose to test a hypothesis, and to implement changes if and only if the hypothesis proves correct. Two points are relevant to experiments. One, the organization needs to ascertain whether the experiment itself meets the relevant criteria outlined earlier, such as those pertaining to costs compared to benefits, fit with the strategic plan, and risks. Two, the organization needs to ascertain what happens if the experiment is successful. Does the proposed change also pass those tests? There is no point in proceeding with an experiment that cannot be implemented even if it works.

Smart Growth

Change in any organization can be painful. It brings costs, risks, uncertainty. People grow accustomed to the usual ways of doing things, and it is hard to get them to do things differently. Positive change achieves results. It enables an organization not just to grow, but to grow in an intelligent fashion. "Smart" growth, rather than growth itself, should be the objective of any health care organization.

Like the police, health care practitioners and administrators have to learn new ways of doing things if their organizations are to survive in the new value-not-volume environment. They thus depend on their ability to inspire and identify projects and initiatives that will lead them in the right direction. As companies in other industries have discovered, innovation is the sine qua non of growth—and it may be the only thing that prevents an organization's premature death. In an environment that is changing as rapidly and as fundamentally as today's, the job of creating and developing the right projects is essential for any organization that wants to succeed.

SUMMARY

- Changes in health care require organizations to take a more active approach than they did in the past. They need to identify, select, and develop the ideas that will make a real difference.

- You can't select the right initiatives without a strategic plan. Initiatives are the method by which an organization pursues its strategic plan.

- Projects that fit the plan can come from a variety of sources, including listening sessions and gemba walks.

- Project ideas need to undergo a concept exploration phase. The concept initiator has to determine whether the idea is worth pursuing and whether it fits with the organization's needs and culture. The initiator can then develop a plan of concept.

NOTES

1. James Q. Wilson, "Hard Times, Fewer Crimes," *Wall Street Journal*, May 28, 2011, http://online.wsj.com/article/SB10001424052702304066504576345553135009870.html.

2. I discuss mission, vision, and values at greater length in chapter 8 of my book: David A. Shore, *The Trust Prescription for Healthcare: Building Your Reputation with Consumers* (Chicago: Health Administration Press, 2005).

3. See Jim Womack, *Gemba Walks* (Boston: Lean Enterprise Institute, 2011).

5

Selecting, Prioritizing, and Monitoring Change Initiatives

Pity the admissions committee at Harvard College, the undergraduate division of Harvard University. More than 34,000 young men and women applied for acceptance to the college's graduating class of 2016. Of these, about half scored 700 or higher (out of a possible 800) on the math Scholastic Aptitude Test (SAT). Nearly as many scored that well on the other two SAT sections, critical reading and writing. About 3,800 applicants ranked number one in their high school class. The vast majority were qualified to do the work at Harvard. However, the college could accept only a little more than 2,000, or about 6 percent of applicants. Talk about selection difficulties.

Medicine has always had selection issues of its own, exemplified by the word *triage*. Triage originated in the First World War, as medical corpsmen and physicians began separating wounded soldiers into three groups: those likely to die regardless of treatment, those who needed immediate treatment, and those whose treatment could be delayed. Today, triage is used by physicians and nurses in clinics and emergency rooms, and by first responders and clinicians at the scene of a disaster. The goal—not so different from during wartime—is to identify patients who require and can benefit from urgent care, as opposed to those who are beyond help and those who can wait for care. The German system of triage, one among many, uses five codes to determine the urgency of treatment: T1 (acute danger for life), T2 (severe injury), T3 (minor or no injury), T4 (no or small chance of survival), and T5 (deceased). Each assessment takes about ninety seconds per patient. The system makes a crucial assumption with important ethical implications: that medical resources in any emergency are going to be limited, and that effort spent on saving someone who is going to die anyway is wasted if it could have been directed to someone else.[1]

All this has a bearing on the issue of selecting the right change initiatives and assigning them relative priority.

The selection and prioritization of change events are difficult because of a confluence of factors. One is that there are so many possible projects. Health care organizations are already swamped with initiatives, and the processes outlined in chapter 4 should produce more rather than fewer ideas for new ones. Like Harvard applicants, many proposals seem worth accepting. Resources and time, however, are limited. In an ideal world, with unlimited quantities of both, the project selection process would be trivial: every seemingly good project could be tried, one after the other. In the real world, no organization can successfully pursue more than a fraction of the initiatives that are proposed to it. In fact, the fewer it pursues, the greater the chance of success with each one. This is a notion that we will revisit later in this chapter.

Organizations thus need a *method* of selecting and prioritizing projects. One can imagine a method that is purely subjective, with a person or group simply deciding which ones they like best. One can also imagine a more objective process, with projects ranked according to some external metric, such as likely return on investment. The ideal, of course, is to combine the best of both worlds: using quantitative methods to remove as much bias as possible, and using qualitative or subjective judgments to ensure that the data are assembled and decisions are made in a practical manner. The art of selecting projects is to accept a good proposal quickly without dismissing a seemingly questionable one too soon.

In this chapter we will examine how health care organizations can do all this: how they can select projects, prioritize them, monitor them as they proceed, and terminate them when necessary. It is a difficult task, akin in principle to that of the Harvard admissions committee or the triage nurse, and in my experience most organizations have not even begun to confront its challenges. But that is no reason to hold back. If health care is to change, organizations will need to undertake this job, and do it right.

THE PROJECT AND PORTFOLIO MANAGEMENT REVIEW BOARD

First and foremost, an organization needs a *mechanism* for selecting, prioritizing, and managing projects. Right now, few organizations have any such mechanism, except for the very largest projects. Typically, no one in the organization approves all projects. No one coordinates them, rank-orders them in terms of the organization's priorities, or measures and reports results. No one monitors these projects across their life cycle, and no one has responsibility for terminating them when they have outlived their usefulness or achieved their ends. This is like an airport without air traffic control, or an organism without a central nervous system. Many of the participants in my classes and executive programs tell me about feeling overwhelmed by the projects they are involved in, and seek guidance from a senior executive. "I have five projects, and I can't get them all done. Which are most important?" the harried staffer asks the vice president. The VP, of course, answers, "All of them"—because she has no way of knowing the answer to the question.

This is why health care organizations need what I call a project and portfolio management review board (PPMRB).

I like this rather cumbersome name because it clearly describes the board's function. Its job is to monitor not just this or that project but the organization's entire portfolio of initiatives. The board establishes a framework for selecting projects. It reviews proposals, approving some and rejecting others, and sending still others back to the concept initiator for more work. It sets priorities. It also reviews projects as they proceed. It monitors their progress, asks for course corrections when necessary, and releases additional resources when a project passes specified milestones successfully. Its job is gatekeeping, tollgating, oversight. When a project has outlived its usefulness, the board serves as judge, jury, and executioner. The board *is* the central nervous system for change events that most health care organizations now lack. It acts as the agent of the executive team, implementing the organization's strategy through projects. The PPMRB thus shares a mission with the organization's board of directors: it seeks to increase the organization's value to all its stakeholders.

Who should be on the board? A well-functioning PPMRB needs to include representatives of three groups:

- **Administrators—but not necessarily the chief executive**. Only rarely does a PPMRB include the CEO. Only rarely does it include more than a single member of the senior leadership team. One top executive—the chief operating officer or the chief financial officer—might volunteer to serve on it. The other members of this subgroup within the PPMRB should include administrators, managers, unit heads, or all three.

- **Clinicians**. Physicians are key stakeholders in virtually all health care organizations. The board should thus include some physician executives, preferably from different specialties. It should also include nurses and other clinicians. The evaluation of many health care projects requires experienced clinical judgment, and only professionals can provide it. Moreover, without physician buy-in, the likelihood that any change event in health care will succeed is unpredictable.

- **Technical specialists and other employees**. A financial specialist should be on the board to help analyze budget requests and monitor financial resources. An IT expert should be on it as well, because these days nearly every project in health care involves IT in one way or another. Depending on the organization and its priorities, the board may need to include technicians or others with specialized expertise.

In general, greater diversity in board membership leads to a wider range of perspectives and greater likelihood of success. Be careful, however, not to make the board too large. A well-functioning board typically involves only ten or twelve people.

I said that the PPMRB is the agent of the organization's executive team. Ultimately it is accountable to the CEO. But this does not mean that the CEO or any other executive who is not on the board should stick a nose into its daily business. Rather, the organization would do well to follow John Carver's method of managing internal relationships, known as policy governance.[2] Under policy governance, the executive team establishes the ends or goals that the board is expected to meet. It then empowers the PPMRB to pursue those ends, with some rules about the methods or means it may use to do so. Of course, it monitors the board's performance along the way. What it does not do is tell the board how to do its job. The PPMRB functions as an autonomous entity as long as it is pursuing the designated ends and not violating the rules about means.

In my view, autonomy of this sort is essential to the PPMRB's successful operation. Board members will quickly develop a great deal of specialized knowledge about the projects in their portfolio. The executive team will lack that detailed knowledge. Board members will become experts in project portfolio management and review; the executive team will lack that level of expertise, and would be likely to complicate matters if it got involved in the process. There are deeper reasons for autonomy as well. Authorship leads to ownership, it is said. If the board feels responsible and accountable for its actions, it will take on that responsibility and accountability willingly. It will "own" its decisions and (in all likelihood) make better ones for precisely that reason.

A review board might sound like a terribly bureaucratic entity, with a thick stack of rule books and procedural guidelines. I have an altogether different conception. A PPMRB is much like a venture capital firm. It invests the organization's resources. It is looking for a payback, sometimes a big one—not always in dollars, to be sure, but in some sort of greater value for the organization's stakeholders. Like a venture capitalist (VC), the board should not fear failure. Indeed, it should expect some of its projects to fail, as projects are the laboratory for change experiments. When one does fail, the PPMRB should act quickly to terminate the project. "Shoot the dogs and chase the winners," the VCs like to say, and however politically incorrect the metaphor, it is a good rule of thumb. The board should get into projects slowly, making sure that every one it approves is a reasonable investment. If the investment goes sour, however, it should exit quickly.

One more comment on the board's overall approach: it needs a designated risk watcher.

A change initiative, after all, is a complex event. It may seem to be succeeding on its own terms while having unintended consequences elsewhere in the system. Or it may fail, with consequences far greater than expected. Health care organizations deal with matters of life and death and cannot afford *any* failure that jeopardizes patient well-being or the smooth functioning of the organization. The risk watcher's job is to identify the outlying possibilities, the risks of unintended consequences or of catastrophic failure. He or she should have a contact—a sort of risk-watch designee—on every project the board approves, and should consult with those contacts regularly. It is critical to the board's overall success that it never be blindsided by risks it has failed to anticipate.

CRITERIA FOR PROJECT SELECTION

Many businesses operate on the principle of selection—and they have someone else do the first round of the process. Publishers, for example, prefer to accept book projects that have been previously vetted by a trusted literary agent. They know that the agent won't send them a proposal unless he or she believes that the book can be successful and that the publisher can do a good job with it. For much of their sales, health insurance companies rely on brokers, who provide them with qualified leads. If the brokers are doing their job well, the prospective clients that they send to an insurance company are much more likely to close a deal than someone who walks in off the street.

The PPMRB is something like an agent or a broker. Acting on behalf of the organization, it selects the projects most likely to succeed, most likely to make a difference, most likely to further the organization's goals. It does this by creating systematic processes that allow it to review all the projects that have been put forward for decision making and action. When the board is created, it reviews existing initiatives. Then it moves on to reviewing newly submitted concepts. It selects projects that meet agreed-on criteria—the first stage gate—and then subjects them to further review, evaluation, and prioritization.

What are these agreed-on criteria? The fundamental one, of course, is consistency with the organization's mission, vision, and values (MV^2). The PPMRB is the enforcer, the guardian, of MV^2. The board will find when it begins operation that many existing projects do not square with MV^2, and it will have to decide what to do about each one. Does the initiative create value in some other way? Can it be reoriented so that it fits better with MV^2? Should it be terminated right now? As for new projects, in theory every idea that comes before the board will fit with MV^2, because the concept initiator has taken mission, vision, and values into account. In practice things are seldom so clear cut, and the board will find itself rejecting many proposals that do not reinforce the organization's MV^2.[3]

Assuming consistency with MV^2, the board must then evaluate projects on other criteria (figure 5.1). Three are particularly important:

- **Necessity**. In this case, the board has no choice but to approve. The initiative may be imposed from the outside by some new regulatory requirement. It may be essential to the functioning—or better functioning—of the organization. People's ideas about what is necessary evolve over time, so an initiative that was nice to have five years ago might today be seen as a need-to-have. Electronic health records, for instance, have in most cases moved from an option to a requirement. And because medicine is constantly evolving, any organization must ensure that it can deliver state-of-the-art treatments in any clinical area on which it focuses.

- **Feasibility.** "Does our organization have the capacity to undertake this project? Are the social capital and financial capital—the skills and the money—readily available? Is the time frame appropriate, given where we are now?" These questions are broad, and the answers will always be partly subjective. But a good proposal will confront them directly and include reasonable answers.

- **Evaluability.** A project that cannot be evaluated is one that can neither succeed nor fail. The PPMRB should make sure that there are methods and mechanisms available to gauge the progress and outcomes of a project. It should look in particular for so-called SMART techniques—specific, measurable, attainable, relevant, and time bound—of evaluation.

In many businesses, the evaluation of a project typically turns on a single variable: projected return on investment (ROI). In health care, ROI may not be the only measure that matters, but it is still important. The PPMRB must consider the ROI of all initiatives, just because every initiative costs money and most are likely to have some effect on the organization's cash flow. The financial representative on the board should take responsibility for seeing that project proposals include net present value analysis or any other financial indicator that may be appropriate. Of course, nothing is ever simple in health care. An organization may decide to undertake a project that has a negative financial ROI because it improves the quality of care or the patient experience. To be sure, such improvements should

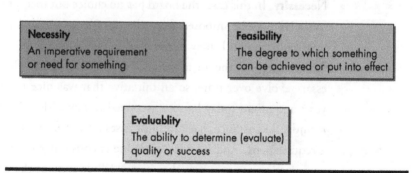

Figure 5.1 Initial Project Evaluation Criteria

ultimately be reflected in more admissions, enhanced reputation, and other variables that eventually will affect the financial statements. But it may be difficult for the board to quantify the financial returns. It should therefore ask for careful experimentation and evaluation before it commits a large amount of resources. *Piloting* is a topic we will revisit shortly.

This brings us to project *size*, a variable that cuts across all of the ones I have just been outlining. Virtually all the data about projects reinforce the famous dictum of the architect Mies van der Rohe: "Less is more." The likelihood of project success is inversely related to project size. The reason isn't hard to fathom: little things are easier to do than big things. Think of the biggest public works project in recent years, Boston's so-called Big Dig. Officially known as the Central Artery/Tunnel Project, the Big Dig recessed a major highway into a tunnel under the city of Boston. (To call it a "project" is a misnomer—it was actually a program, an entire portfolio of projects—but bear with me.) The Big Dig took years longer than expected and ran billions of dollars over its budget. Even at this writing, long after the project's completion, Massachusetts state officials continue to find parts of the Big Dig that were completed poorly or improperly.

Staying within the scope of a project means delivering on the project's ambitions—no less, but (more important) no more. It suggests a "lean ethic" for projects, whereby proposals set out modest ambitions and try to achieve them with as little wasted time and as few squandered resources as possible. Though this book is primarily about launching and leading rather than implementing projects, it is worth noting that my model, the Project Activation and Management System (PAMS), typically cuts the size of project teams by 40 to 50 percent, just by splitting contributors into *domain experts*, who are core team members, and *subject matter advisers*, who are available only when needed. Leanness of this sort needs to be built into the plan of concept itself, and the PPMRB should insist on it.

Typically, the board will require that any large project be piloted—that is, tried out on a small scale first. If a pilot fails, it is a pretty good sign that the project as a whole is poorly conceived, and piloting has enabled the organization to avoid wasting a lot of time and money on it. At the very least, the results of the pilot may suggest project plan revisions. If the pilot succeeds, it *may* be worth taking the next step. But be careful! It is common for a pilot to succeed and for the initiative to fail as soon as it is scaled up. The organization may want to try one pilot and then another in a different area, or a small pilot first and a larger one next. Scaling an initiative nearly always brings challenges of its own, and a single pilot may not be sufficient to indicate what they are.

Piloting is not the only condition a PPMRB may place on the projects it reviews. Indeed, there are many different outcomes possible for every proposal coming before the board (see figure 5.2). It may approve the proposal with certain conditions. These conditions usually will be easy to meet—for

Used to organize and prioritize the ideas for improvement that have been mentioned in the improvement opportunity hopper		
	(I) Implement	**(C) Challenge**
	*High impact *Big payoff *Easy to do/implement	*High impact *Big payoff *Hard to do/implement
	(P) Possible	**(K) Kibosh/crush**
	*Low impact *Small payoff *Easy to do/implement	*Low impact *Small payoff *Hard to do/implement
Considerations		
Impact:	Low ⟵⟶ High	
	*Quality of patient care *Patient safety *Current performance measures *Value added work *Timeliness/access (e.g., Decrease patient or staff wait times for information, supplies, or each other, etc.)	
Implementation:	Easier ⟵⟶ Harder	
	*Cost *Timeline (e.g., ≤ 14 days is easy, and ≥ 15 days is harder) *Resources (e.g., Need for equipment or supplies, human capital, etc.)	

Figure 5.2 Prioritization PICK Chart

Source: Adapted from Kim Carli, Accelerating City of Hope Excellence, City of Hope National Medical Center.

example, the board might require that the project make itself more "green" by using energy-efficient materials. Then, too, the board might return the proposal with a request for recalibration and resubmission. The changes requested in this case would usually be larger, requiring the concept initiator to rework his or her idea. For instance, the board might request that the project be scaled down to make its budget fit more easily with the organization's funding capabilities. The board might even request that the initiator break the project down into more manageable chunks and submit each one for separate approval. All such decisions are consistent with a good board's interest in keeping its ventures as small and as manageable as possible. No health care organization can afford the equivalent of a Big Dig.

A winning plan of concept, incidentally, does not need to be fully fleshed out. It can be little more than a carefully developed concept, with a plan for piloting or other testing. The PPMRB, in approving this kind of proposal, should not approve an entire budget all at once. Rather, it can set aside resources for research, design, development, testing, and eventual rollout. A seasoned concept initiator will include a budget that requests specific amounts for each stage. That enables the PPMRB to plan for funding should the proposal turn out to be worth supporting through all of its various stages.

One more general comment: though most health care organizations do not have anything like the PPMRB that I am proposing, some do have a process in place to select projects. In that case, the job is to strengthen that process, and to score project proposals against a generally accepted standardized framework. Organizations in this position have a great advantage in that they aren't creating something wholly from scratch, but rather can build on what is already in place.

To sum up: just as a concept initiator can make use of a list of early questions (see chapter 4), the PPMRB might want to put a list of selection criteria up on its bulletin board. The following, adapted from the research firm Gartner Group, is one possible set of criteria that touches on the points I have mentioned:[4]

- **Strategic alignment**—How well does the initiative align with MV^2 and the long-term strategic goals of the organization?

- **Process impact**—To what extent would the project require changes in existing business or clinical processes?

- **Technical considerations**—How scalable and resilient is the project? How simple would it be to integrate the project with existing processes and structures?

- **Direct and indirect payback**—What benefits will the initiative produce in terms of better patient care, better experiences, improved safety, cost savings, additional revenue, or other indicators?

- **Risk**—How likely is it that the initiative will fail to meet expectations or have unintended consequences, and what are the probable costs of both?

The plan of concept details additional items, such as the initiative's necessity and feasibility. A PPMRB that can answer these questions about each proposal is well on its way to selecting the projects that are right for the organization.

PRIORITIZING PROJECTS

If selection is the first stage gate, then prioritization is the second, because the fact is, few organizations can undertake all the good, important, potentially beneficial ideas that come their way. They rarely have the financial resources, and they almost never have enough people with the necessary skills. So they can pursue only a fraction of the proposals they receive.

I would take this indisputable truth one step farther. Organizations should undertake only a small number of initiatives at any one time. They should "shrink to manage."

After all, what happens when there are a large number of projects under way? The situation stretches the organization's capacity for change. It asks too much of people, both those who are involved in the initiatives and those who are affected. Projects begin colliding with each other, yet the organization is often unaware of the cumulative impact. The sheer volume of endeavors is in many instances a leading cause of failure, because many projects get lost in the shuffle. They wind up as orphans, involving lots of people but belonging to nobody.

How much better, then, to have only a few well-defined and well-understood initiatives? All will receive the support they deserve. None will get lost. The individuals involved will not feel so stressed, either by the work they are putting in or by the possibility that their work lives will have to change. It is obviously far more effective for an organization to launch five great projects than to launch fifteen mediocre ones. But the corollary is equally true and often less appreciated: it is far more effective to launch five great projects than to launch fifteen great projects, because the fifteen are less likely to remain great.

In any event, what could be more fundamental than deciding what are the most important initiatives to undertake right now, given the organization's situation and needs? That is what prioritization does. The problem is, prioritization is hard.

Take what may be the most famous historical situation involving prioritization: getting passengers from the *Titanic* into lifeboats. The order came out: "Women and children in and lower away." One officer took the order to mean women and children first. Another decided that it meant women and children only.[5] Embedded in that seemingly noble objective, indeed, was a morass of ambiguity and contradiction. What about a single male widower traveling with his child? Should the widower be saved at the expense of a childless woman? Should he be rejected, thus risking making the child an orphan? And how should the crew have prioritized the women and children who *were* allowed into the lifeboats? Crew members on the *Titanic* soon realized that they had an extremely poor prioritization process. In the event, the odds of a first-class female passenger's surviving were many times greater than the odds of survival for a steerage-class woman.

How can an organization effectively prioritize its projects? It obviously needs an agreed-on method to compare every one with the others.

Quadrants

One of the simplest methods of prioritization involves Stephen R. Covey's four quadrants. In Covey's formulation—elaborated in his self-help classic, *The 7 Habits of Highly Effective People*—there is a simple two-by-two matrix, with "Important" along the y- or vertical axis and "Urgent" along the x- or horizontal axis or top.[6] You assign tasks to one of the four quadrants: Q1 (important and urgent), Q2 (important but not urgent), Q3 (urgent but not important), and Q4 (neither urgent nor important). Covey assumed that Q1 activities would take care of themselves—you couldn't avoid them—and emphasized the importance of focusing your attention on Q2 activities, those that are important but not urgent. When we ignore Q2 activities, he argued, they will eventually become Q1, and soon we will find ourselves putting out fires that never need have ignited. Proactive tackling of Q2 tasks gives us a sense of control over our lives. Spending time on Q3 or even Q4 tasks may give us the illusion of getting things done, but more often than not our accomplishments will consist of doing the wrong things well. Many Q2 tasks, in contrast, are critical but not immediately obvious. They are important, but because they are not urgent we are unaware of the need to do them. Seeking out these tasks helps us stay one step ahead of the game.

There's a vital parallel between Covey's Q2 and the idea of medical prevention. Triage that operates purely according to the urgency of patients' need for care is a defensive, reactive approach to health care. The triage mentality, which pervades much of health care, is essentially what Covey would call Q1 thinking, that is, doing things only when they become urgent. But the ongoing transformation of health care redefines the concept of triage. Patient treatment should be prioritized according to a farsighted evaluation of everything that is urgent now *as well as everything that may become urgent in the future if left untreated.* This is preventive medicine at its best. It does not require us to abandon the notion of triage, but it does require that we expand our criteria for the sorting of patients. It is a proactive kind of triage, tackling the important before it becomes urgent. It provides a useful model for thinking about projects.

Another helpful two-by-two model is the so-called PICK chart, developed at Lockheed Martin. PICK stands for possible, implement, challenge, and kibosh/crush. In this case the quadrants are labeled according to the impact of the project on the one hand and the difficulty of implementation on the other. The considerations affecting an initiative's impact might include its effect on patient care and safety; on current performance measures (including financial ones); and on the patient experience (for example, access, or the feeling of being cared for). Considerations affecting difficulty of implementation might include cost; the overall timeline; and the need for nonfinancial resources, such as people's time (figure 5.2).

Of course, one can pack additional information into one's charts, to help everyone on the board grasp some of the relative costs and benefits of a proposed project portfolio. Figure 5.3 shows a very useful "bubble chart," with benefit to the organization ranked on the y-axis, difficulty of implementation ranked on the x-access, and the size of each bubble representing the associated project's cost. One may even want to color in the bubbles to indicate the category of project being considered in each instance. I have found that management tends to appreciate receiving such graphical representations of complex information.

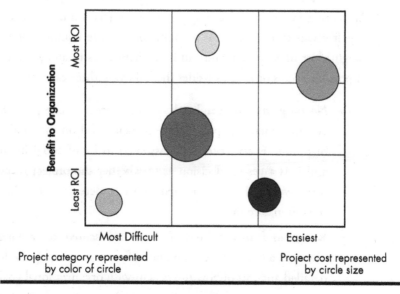

Figure 5.3 Project Portfolio Bubble Chart

Source: Adapted from Eric Verzuh and Ralph Kliem, "Project Portfolio Management: Align Project Resources with Business Strategy," February 19, 2001, http://www.mpug.com/articles/project-portfolio-management-align-project-resources-with-business-strategy/.

Payoff versus time

In this method, the PPMRB gives each project a rating by dividing the expected payoff by the amount of time and resources required to achieve it. The idea is that the project with the highest payoff that takes the least time and resources should be done first.

The payoff derives from a formula that incorporates subjective ratings based on several factors, which might include patient safety, clinical outcomes, importance to the customer, feasibility or likelihood of success (risk), financial returns, and leverage (positive impact on other processes). The denominator—time—is calculated by incorporating financial cost and person hours required into a single variable.

Other scoring models

All scoring models involve assigning each project a numerical score. The payoff-versus-time method is a simple one. More complex ones can be weighted or unweighted, and can limit themselves to an agreed-on range of possible scores or not. Consider the following three examples:

- **No range and unweighted**. A project receives one point for each criterion met, and projects are chosen based on the total number of points. Every criterion is assumed to be of equal importance, and it is a yes-no decision as to whether the project meets it. In other words, there is no opportunity to determine to what extent the criteria are met.

- **Range and unweighted**. Projects are scored on a range—for example, a Likert scale from one to five. This option provides more detailed analysis of how projects fit with organizational goals.

- **Range and weighted**. In addition to scoring criteria on a range, this option provides a weighted score for each criterion, indicating how important each consideration is. This scoring model offers a more robust analysis of how well projects fit with organizational priorities.

In creating weighted scoring models, organizations obviously need to determine how much value to assign to each of their top priorities. These weights do not need to be set in stone. As a company refocuses its objectives over time, calculations for weighting measures may be modified to fit with current goals. And given the dynamic environment in which health care organizations operate, they may need to revisit scoring values and criteria on a regular basis. Further, they may need to make changes to ensure that the weighting system keeps up with changing priorities in the marketplace as well as in the organization.

With the scoring methodology established and potential projects rated according to a set of criteria and their weighted values, organizations can prioritize projects based on that methodology. High-strategy, high-return, low-risk projects will generally be seen as high priority. This helps ensure that the right projects are green-lighted based on relatively objective criteria. When a proposed project receives a score below the cutoff line, the organization must consider declining the project.

Whatever the prioritization approach, it should be rational and transparent, and linked to the organization's strategic goals. The prioritization process will thus reflect the organization's MV^2. Bear in mind that the prioritization of projects only represents the order in which they are to be launched; it says nothing about the care and attention to be dedicated to each. The lowest-priority item in the queue is simply the one that is to be done last, sequentially. It is not the one that is the least important or the one that can be done with the least care. Prioritization is simply an ordering of events, not a listing of importance. In the clinical setting, every event is important. The right prioritization is an ordering that maximizes the benefit, but it is contingent on everything's being completed thoroughly and successfully.

What must be avoided at all costs is the all-too-common laissez-faire approach to projects within health care organizations—that is, implementing them without considering resource allocation, overall importance, or competing projects. Prioritization is essential, both to achieve organizational objectives and to minimize risk.

MONITORING PROJECTS

The PPMRB's job is not simply to review, approve, and prioritize projects. That gets projects started. But unless someone is constantly monitoring them, the organization will wind up back where it started, with too many projects and too little attention paid to them.

Monitoring includes a variety of tasks, including the following:

- **Tracking progress.** Every initiative needs to be tracked as it proceeds toward its objectives. Board members should meet with project implementation leaders, project sponsors, or both, perhaps at every milestone, to assess accomplishments, review upcoming plans, and discuss potential obstacles and challenges. Board meetings should include brief discussions of every project. A chart on the wall with green, yellow, and red "stoplight" indicators can show respectively which projects are on track, which are encountering challenges, and which have run into apparently insuperable obstacles.

- **Approving next-stage resource allocation.** Most projects of any size will include a series of stages, marked by the achievement of specific milestones. It is the board's job to evaluate whether the project has indeed achieved its milestones and, if it has, to approve additional phased funding or whatever else may be required in the next stage.

- **Decommissioning a failed project.** This is an essential part of the PPMRB's mandate. Projects proliferate today because no one discontinues failing and failed projects. Every failed project deserves death with dignity, including a termination meeting that thanks team members for their efforts and a "lessons learned" session that captures and records the reasons for the project's failure.

The board's oversight enables an organization to move beyond the situation—all too common today—in which once a project is approved, no one looks at it again. It enables the organization to avoid throwing good money after bad.

The board also should *rebalance the project portfolio* periodically.

In their periodic review sessions, board members need to examine every project to see whether it still makes sense. The initiative may be proceeding merrily on its way; it may even be achieving some of its milestones. But if it would no longer be approved in light of the organization's goals, it is a potential waste of resources and should be terminated. This is often a difficult step for a board to take, because the project team may not agree that its endeavors no longer have a high priority. But it is an essential one. Unless the board periodically prunes the project tree, it will be a poor manager of the organization's resources.

There is another objective that is also involved in rebalancing the project portfolio. Looking at all the projects together allows the board to spot imbalances. It may have inadvertently approved too many large projects. It may have approved too many projects in the same area, or too many that carry a significant measure of risk. Conversely, all of its projects may be safe, low-payoff enterprises, with none of the high-risk, high-reward variety. Like the venture capitalists they essentially are, board members need appropriate balances of investment sizes, kinds of projects, and riskiness.

• • •

Nearly everyone who works in health care can remember being involved in projects that did not turn out as hoped. Sometimes the fault lies with poor project management. Far more often, the trouble was built in from the beginning. The project was poorly conceived, poorly planned, or inadequately resourced. It never received an evaluation from critical reviewers—reviewers who could have helped strengthen it. It had no appropriate stage gates, so team members set out on a long journey without the help of any landmarks or milestones along the way. If you have been in this situation, you know the frustrations. It is hard to avoid the conclusion that you have been wasting your time, and by extension the organization's resources. The next time someone asks you to volunteer for a project, you will be less likely to agree.

Such a situation is equally troublesome from the standpoint of a health care organization. People in the organization are trying hard to get things done, and yet the organization does not seem to advance toward its goals. MV^2 remains a piece of paper on the boardroom wall; it is not a living, breathing reality. There is no sense of progress. The organization's resources are being misused, wasted, or both.

A formal process of project review and launch, institutionalized in a well-functioning PPMRB, can fix this problem. The board selects the right projects, nurtures them, watches over them, and pulls the plug when necessary. It creates a portfolio of projects that waste no one's time, and that move the organization in the direction of its strategic objectives. Instead of building in failure from the beginning, it builds in success.

SUMMARY

- Organizations need a systematic method of selecting and prioritizing change initiatives. The key is the creation of a project and portfolio management review board.

- The board should include administrators, clinicians, technical specialists, and other employees as appropriate. It needs a designated risk watcher, whose job it is to watch out for dangers and pitfalls.

- Criteria for project selection include consistency with the organization's mission, vision, and values (MV^2); necessity (mandates); feasibility; and evaluability.

- In general, smaller projects are better than big ones. Pilots are often a good way of approaching larger projects.

- The board should systematically prioritize projects according to agreed-on criteria. It should also monitor projects—tracking their progress, approving next-stage resource allocation, and decommissioning failed projects when necessary.

NOTES

1. Michael Bayeff-Filloff, "Analysis of the Incidence and Causes of Mass Casualty Events in a Southern Germany Medical Rescue Area," *Unfallchirurg* 105 (November 2002): 968–973.
2. See John Carver, *Boards That Make a Difference: A New Design for Leadership in Non-profit and Public Organizations*, 3rd ed. (Hoboken, NJ: Wiley, 2006).
3. For those interested in more information on the role and importance of mission, vision, and values, please see David A. Shore, *The Trust Prescription for Healthcare: Building Your Reputation with Consumers* (Chicago: Health Administration Press, 2005).
4. Tony Murphy, *Achieving Business Value from Technology* (Hoboken, NJ: Wiley, 2002).
5. See David Gleicher, *The Rescue of the Third Class on the Titanic: A Revisionist History*, Research in Maritime History 31 (St. John's, Newfoundland: International Maritime Economic History Association, 2006).
6. Stephen R. Covey, *The 7 Habits of Highly Effective People: Powerful Lessons for Personal Change* (1990; repr., New York: Free Press, 2004).

PART 3

Choose the Right People

INTRODUCTION: HOW IMPORTANT ARE DECISIONS ABOUT PEOPLE?

Anyone who thinks seriously about change initiatives in health care quickly runs into a conundrum. Is it the people who matter most, or is it the processes? Is the most important thing to get personnel decisions right—or are those decisions essentially irrelevant, with establishing great processes being what really counts?

This is no idle dispute, because it reflects a great debate taking place not only in health care but also in management generally.

On one side are the process advocates. Consider the point of view of Fujio Cho, who at this writing is chairman of Toyota Motor Corporation: "At Toyota we get brilliant results from average people managing a brilliant process. Others get average results from brilliant people managing broken processes."[1]

There is no doubt in Cho's mind about which is more important. The great management theorist Peter Drucker seemingly agreed: "No institution can possibly survive if it needs geniuses or supermen to manage it. It must be organized in such a way as to be able to get along under a leadership composed of average human beings."[2]

In health care, the Institute of Medicine's famous 1999 report *To Err Is Human*—which charged that up to ninety-eight thousand people a year were dying unnecessarily because of medical errors—laid the blame squarely on processes. "Errors are not caused by bad people," it said, "but by bad systems."[3] The actor Dennis Quaid echoed this analysis. Quaid became a nationally known advocate for patient safety following a harrowing family experience in 2007. His twelve-day-old twins developed an infection, and he and his wife brought them to a Los Angeles hospital. There, the twins nearly died when they accidently received one thousand times the intended dose of the drug heparin, an anticoagulant. In 2012 Quaid, who is himself a licensed pilot, wrote an article in the *Journal of Patient Safety* with Captain Chesley "Sully" Sullenberger, the pilot who became a national hero when he successfully landed a disabled U.S. Airways flight 1599 in the Hudson River, and two other coauthors, both with aviation experience. The article argued for the application of aviation safety practices to medicine. "We don't have bad people," the authors wrote, "we have bad systems."[4]

Health care professionals have spent a great deal of effort in recent years attempting to improve their systems. A systems approach is, after all, the foundation of evidence-based medicine: physicians who systematically follow best clinical practices for a given condition will achieve better results on average than those who rely on their own experience, no matter how talented they may be as individuals. It's the system that counts, not the person. One of America's most respected health care institutions, Seattle's Virginia Mason Medical Center, has embraced the systems approach wholeheartedly. It adopted the fundamentals of the Toyota Production System, renaming it the Virginia Mason Production System, and translated its precepts to a health care environment. "Our Virginia Mason Production System is methodically removing every barrier between you and perfect patient care," says the center's website.[5] In Wisconsin, the four-hospital system Thedacare has also been drawing on the principles of Toyota-style lean manufacturing to improve care and reduce costs. Among its accomplishments is a drop in the mortality rate for coronary bypass surgery from 4 percent to 1.4 percent and then to 0 percent. Meanwhile, "a [coronary] patient's average time spent in the hospital fell from 6.3 days to 4.9, and costs for a coronary bypass declined 22 percent."[6]

So systems are clearly important. But let us look for a moment at the other side of the debate: those who emphasize the importance of people. A series of studies and reports from McKinsey & Company argued that the most important corporate resource over the next two decades will be talent. According to McKinsey, given the right kind of culture, talented people have better ideas than others, and they execute those ideas better. Even if organizations have plenty of good ideas and plenty of money, they may not have enough talented people to execute those ideas. McKinsey pointed to companies, such as General Electric, Home Depot, and others, that have made a point of attracting and developing top talent. To be sure, the fact that one of the firm's studies included Enron as an exemplar does not exactly help the case. But the other positive examples remain strong.

McKinsey-style arguments for the primacy of people have a long and distinguished history. Harvard and other elite universities have long sought out the most respected academics to add to their faculty. Many elite hospitals and medical centers have pursued a similar strategy: get the best people, and the quality will take care of itself. Lo and behold, Drucker himself weighed in on this side of the debate: the most important decisions any executive makes, he said, are decisions about people, because those decisions will determine the performance capacity of the organization.[7]

Nor is this approach limited to the United States. In 2012 I was able to teach a program to health care leaders in the Persian Gulf nation of Qatar, which had recently established a "national vision" for the year 2030. The vision rested on four pillars, one of which was the idea that "people are a country's most valuable assets." Part of the vision was a national health strategy, which identified one essential requirement for success: "Human resources are the most critical prerequisites. The first step in implementation is identifying the human resources that will be responsible for the outcome."[8] Qatar is changing, and its leaders have determined that the key ingredient of successful change is to have—and to invest in—the right people.

Let us sort through this debate as it applies to change initiatives, because each side obviously has merit. The apparent conflict is simply a result of trying to use a single argument like a blanket to cover all possible situations.

Systems manage an organization's ongoing business. No organization could exist without well-established systems and processes for getting things done. And there is little doubt in anyone's mind these days that most systems in health care could be improved. That is really the point of the change initiatives and projects we are discussing in this book: systems improvement. Virginia Mason has embarked on a major program encompassing dozens and dozens of individual projects, each one designed to eliminate waste, reduce costs, improve quality, and achieve the other aims of the Toyota Production System. The result, one hopes, will be an overarching system that minimizes medical errors, maximizes quality of care, and optimizes costs. It will encompass hundreds of subsystems, in each unit and department of the organization. Any organization, of course, needs the best people it can get—but every organization will have to make do with people who have human flaws and failings. The point of a system is to minimize the impact of these flaws and failings on the organization's work product—in this case, the care of sick and injured patients and the prevention of illness. Toyota and Virginia Mason are right to emphasize the importance of systems.

This book isn't about the systems that manage an organization's ongoing work. It is about initiatives and projects that *change* an organization. These projects are very likely to involve designing new systems and procedures. They are about moving from a current state to a better state, or from a current system to a better one. They are about innovation. And the only entity that can innovate is a human being. People will design the goals of these projects. They will launch the projects. They will—or will not—be successful. It matters a great deal who those people are: what skills and experience they possess; how they are assembled; and how they become a passionate, committed project team. The chapters in this part of the book will examine each of these topics in detail. They will provide you with a road map for the second great "right" in our approach: selecting the right people. To be successful, change events must involve the right people, not just whoever happens to be available and is willing to say yes when asked to participate.

There is also another way to look at this systems-versus-people dichotomy. Part 2 of this book in effect outlined a system for choosing change initiatives. That system is an essential element in getting projects right. If you don't have a rationale to determine which initiatives to undertake, you will forever be trying to do the wrong things. Part 3 of the book, which begins here, focuses on finding the people who can actually implement this system. And because what we are talking about is creating new systems, the caliber of the people you select is critically important.

In the end, therefore, the conundrum explored in this introduction presents a false dichotomy. A health care organization doesn't need great people *or* great systems. It needs great people *and* great systems, and nowhere are both elements more important than in the selection and launching of change initiatives and projects. In today's project-centric world, the ability of an organization's people to launch and lead change initiatives will more and more determine success in what is now a brutally competitive and fast-changing marketplace.

SUMMARY

- Systems are important, and chapter 5 outlined a system for selecting and prioritizing projects.

- Ultimately, however, people will have to staff that system. Choosing the right people for your initiatives may be the most important set of decisions determining their success.

NOTES

1. Art Kliener, "Leaning towards Utopia," *Strategy+Business* 39 (July 2005): 2–12.
2. Peter F. Drucker, *Concept of the Corporation* (1969; repr., Piscataway, NJ: Transaction Publishers, 1993), 26.
3. Institute of Medicine, *To Err Is Human: Building a Safer Health System* (Washington, DC: National Academies Press, November 1999), http://www.iom.edu/~/media/Files /Report%20Files/1999/To-Err-is-Human/To%20Err%20is%20Human%201999 %20%20report%20brief.pdf.
4. Charles R. Denham et al., "An NTSB for Health Care—Learning from Innovation: Debate and Innovate or Capitulate," *Journal of Patient Safety* 8 (March 2012): 5.
5. See https://www.virginiamason.org/VMPS.
6. John Toussaint, "Writing the New Playbook for U.S. Health Care: Lessons from Wisconsin," *Health Affairs* 28, no. 5 (September–October 2009): 1345, doi: 10.1377 /hlthaff.28.5.1343.
7. Peter F. Drucker, *Managing the Non-Profit Organization* (1990; repr., New York: HarperBusiness, 2006), 145.
8. Supreme Council of Health, State of Qatar, *National Health Strategy 2011–2016: Caring for the Future Executive Summary* (Doha, Qatar: Supreme Council of Health, State of Qatar), 24, accessed March 5, 2013, http://www.nhsq.info/app/media/14.

6

What You Are Looking For

Pity the health care leader charged with finding people to lead and staff a new change initiative. The task of getting the *right* people, as we will shortly see, is hard enough. But he or she must first determine whether *any* people are available. At least five organizational factors are likely to interfere.

One is simply supply and demand. The demand for people to work on projects in health care organizations typically outstrips supply, sometimes by a factor of ten to one. There is a constant need for project teams, just because every organization these days is trying so hard to change. But the supply of people is fixed, at least in the short term. And no administrator or human resources manager wants to go out and hire more bodies, particularly if the only job description available is "Work on projects."

A second, related factor is whether individuals on an organization's staff have the bandwidth to work on projects at all. Everybody in a health care organization has a day job, and some of these jobs are among the most demanding on the planet. To be sure, everybody's job description is likely to include that catch-all phrase, "Other duties as assigned." But in the real world, people are likely to balk at taking on extra assignments—particularly when they feel barely able to get their regular work done in a timely and efficient manner.

A third factor, also related, is the organization's ability to backfill. If half a dozen people are named to a project team—and if the project is complex, strategically important, and thus time consuming—those individuals are likely to spend a significant fraction of their workdays on tasks related to the project. Who will fill in for them at their respective day jobs? An organization needs a great deal of bench strength if it is to embark on serious change initiatives. Health care organizations know the importance of bench strength when it comes to nursing, because a nursing station or shift cannot go uncovered. Most need to learn its importance when it comes to change initiatives.

A fourth factor is matrix conflict. Anybody asked to be on a project team already has a supervisor or manager, to whom he or she is accountable. Once assigned to the project implementation team, the employee now has a project implementation leader, to whom he or she is also accountable. On an organization chart, the member has "solid line" responsibility to the regular boss and "dotted line" responsibility to the project implementation leader. Here, too, the real world intrudes, because it is seldom as simple as an organization chart. People in this situation wonder where their loyalties should lie. They worry about provoking a backlash if they prioritize one set of responsibilities over the other.

Finally there is the issue that we might call "projectus interruptus." Say that a typical initiative lasts for nine months. During that time, some people in any organization will depart for a new position somewhere else. Others will change jobs internally or go on leave. Large organizations learn to cope with such disruptions. It is much harder for a small team working on a demanding change initiative to do so. They cannot afford to have people leave midstream.

At most organizations, these factors are not insurmountable. They are just obstacles to be dealt with, and it is essential that leaders responsible for selecting project teams and project implementation leaders be aware of all of them. But then comes a still more daunting task: leaders must figure out what kind of people they are looking for. Though what I have to say in this chapter applies in some measure to all members of a change team, it applies above all to the initiative's leader, who is the linchpin that will ultimately determine the project's likelihood of success.

The main topic is that time-honored duality, *will* and *skill*, which I will recast slightly as *soft skills* versus *hard skills*.

HARD AND SOFT SKILLS

The year was 2004. David Fox had recently become president of Advocate Good Samaritan Hospital in Downers Grove, Illinois, not far from Chicago. Up to that point, Good Samaritan had hired people the way most organizations do, by looking for exceptional technical skills and relevant experience. The hospital found many such employees, and the staff was highly competent. Not surprisingly, however, there was a great deal of variation in staff members' attitudes, orientation toward service, ability to work in teams, compassion for patients, and commitment to the organization's new vision of providing an exceptional patient experience. How could it be any different? These were all ordinary human beings, and they had been hired for their technical abilities, not for their attitudes.

Fox changed that. He wanted Good Samaritan to embark on a journey "from good to great," and he knew that the trip would require a workforce that expected to be far more engaged and committed than it was in the past. Like leaders at Southwest Airlines and some other forward-looking companies, he and his team began screening first for people with the right attitudes, those whose personality would fit with the emerging Good Samaritan culture. The hospital required appropriate technical skills, of course. But if a candidate wasn't seen as a good fit, he or she was unlikely to be hired. Candidates with the necessary training and experience can learn new technical skills, Fox and his team believed. Candidates with the wrong personality and attitudes, however, are unlikely to metamorphose into enthusiastic, communicative, service-oriented team players.

So it is with change events. In selecting project implementation leaders and staffing project teams, you need, more than anything else, individuals with the right attitudes and the right interpersonal abilities—the "soft" skills, as distinct from the "hard" skills needed to undertake such tasks as scheduling, workflow management, and budgeting.

In focusing on the importance of soft skills, I do not mean to denigrate the importance of technical expertise. Technical expertise is the ticket to entry, the foundation for everything else. Good Samaritan wasn't hiring any nursing school dropouts for RN positions or substandard surgeons for the coronary care unit, no matter how positive those individuals' attitudes might have been. And no project team can hope to succeed unless its leaders and many of its members possess all the technical skills the initiative requires, including experience in project management.

This is no small matter. Physicians, it has been estimated, spend up to 40,000 hours in postsecondary education and training before they become fully fledged doctors. Lawyers don't become partners in a firm until they have at least several years' experience under their belt. Newly hired pilots at major airlines typically have about 4,000 hours of flight experience. They start as flight engineers or first officers; promotion to captain can take another five to fifteen years and is often offered according to seniority. Project management, too, has its professional training. To apply for certification as a Project Management Professional (PMP), a credential offered by the Project Management Institute, a college-educated applicant must have three years of project management experience, at least 4,500 hours of leading and directing projects, and 35 hours of project management education.[1] The difference here is that *every* doctor and lawyer has that advanced training. Of the estimated twenty million individuals who engage in some form of project management, only about one million have had any formal training.[2]

What are the hard skills required? They vary from one project to another. A financial project may require accounting skills, an IT project computer skills, a clinical project medical skills. The project implementation leader must excel at the tasks mentioned earlier: scheduling, workflow management, budgeting, and so on. Project implementation leaders need to know their way around a Gantt chart or a PERT (program evaluation and review technique) chart, and they must be able to use project management software. A leader may also need to be a subject matter expert. You would not want a physician overseeing a project to revamp a medical center's financial systems (though a physician might well serve on the project team). And the leader should have experience managing projects. Green or untested project implementation leaders can start small, with simpler initiatives; only later, when they have proven their mettle, should they be entrusted with bigger or more complex change events.

All that said, the soft skills are ultimately more important to a project's success than pure technical expertise. This truth is coming to be recognized in the wider world of project management. Dave Zielinski, writing in *Training* magazine, reported on the change in 2005:

> If you had asked project-management gurus five years ago to name the most important competencies project managers should have, most would have said technical skills. Today they'd be more inclined to place communications or negotiations acumen at the top of their lists. . . There's no denying the importance of technical expertise to successfully orchestrating a project. Managing an initiative's scope, cost, risk, resources and schedule are all essential skills. Indeed, the quality of up-front planning—and a project leader's skill at replanning as project conditions change—can determine a project's fate all on its own. But in rethinking skill hierarchies, many companies have come to view these more as baseline competencies. Now they regard soft skills . . . such as communication, negotiation, conflict management and persuasion, as higher-order skills.[3]

Why are soft skills so important? Think for a moment about the typical project manager's situation. Project managers do not have a stable base of power. They operate outside of the traditional functional structure. They rarely have the authority to conduct formal performance evaluations or reviews of the people who serve on their project team.[4] Project managers thus are unable to provide many of the conventional inducements of management. If they aren't politically astute and socially adept, nothing good will happen.

Soft skills are even more important in health care. The field has too many surgeons with a terrible bedside manner, too many administrators who are great fund-raisers but who ignore the patient experience. It's an arena in which technical expertise alone is inadequate. Moreover, because we are focusing on health care, I do not limit myself to the conventional list of soft skills. A positive attitude and an upbeat personality are important, to be sure. So are communication skills, enthusiasm, an ability to get along with others, and an ability to work productively on teams, among others. But the environment in a medical center or any other health care organization is more demanding than elsewhere. It isn't just that health care is an unusually complex industry, involving a rare combination of sophisticated technology and high-touch, hands-on interaction. It is also that more is at stake. The rewards of success and the costs of failure are far higher than in most endeavors. Success requires a different and in some ways unique set of soft skills.

We will look at three such skills in this chapter. I think of them as (1) the ability to hold *crucial conversations;* (2) the combination of attributes that Daniel Goleman has called *emotional intelligence;* and (3) the ability to *trust* and to engender trust. If you can find people with these skills, in my experience, the chances that your project will accomplish its objectives on time and on budget will increase by an order of magnitude.

CRUCIAL CONVERSATIONS

Have you had "the Conversation"? This is the question that Pulitzer Prize–winning columnist Ellen Goodman and the Institute for Healthcare Improvement would like all of us to be able to answer in the affirmative.

This particular Conversation, with a capital *C*, has to do with end-of-life choices. Imagine that your elderly mother is dying in a hospital, unable to communicate clearly. The medical professionals want to know the family's wishes. Family members are uncertain. Do they ask for a feeding tube? Do they want a ventilator to help their mother breathe? Should they ask for morphine to control her pain, even if it might hasten her death? *What would she want us to do?* That is always the question on everyone's mind, but, most of the time, the family does not know. They have never talked about it, and now, perhaps, they cannot agree. This is a widespread problem. In Canada, for example—a nation that has studied these situations—an estimated 70 percent of people have no living will setting out their end-of-life wishes. Only 47 percent have designated someone to make end-of-life decisions on their behalf. Fewer than half have spoken to a family member about end-of-life care.

Goodman was an architect of the Conversation Project, which alerts medical professionals and laypeople to the importance of having this conversation well before that final hospital stay. Without it, she and her colleagues point out, we all run the risk of not getting the care we want or else getting care that we do not want. The project's goal is that everyone's end-of-life wishes be expressed and respected.

For this book's purposes, however, we are interested in a different issue: *Why* do we not hold such conversations with our loved ones, given the fact that we are all going to die and that many of us will inevitably endure a prolonged end-of-life illness? The reason, of course, is that such conversations are difficult. They are awkward and sometimes embarrassing. They force us to confront things that we would rather not think about.

Physicians have difficult conversations with patients all the time. An internist must tell some patients that they are suffering from a serious illness. A surgeon must inform some patients that an operation was not successful. A hospitalist must tell some families that their father or mother is not likely to last the night. Surprisingly, though, neither physicians nor members of any other group working in health care settings are particularly good at another kind of crucial conversation, those involving their colleagues. A 2006 study by the American Association of Critical-Care Nurses and the consulting firm VitalSmarts reported that 84 percent of physicians had seen coworkers taking shortcuts that could be dangerous to patients, and 88 percent said they worked with people who showed poor clinical judgment. Yet fewer than 10 percent of physicians, nurses, and other clinical staff said that they directly confronted their colleagues about their concerns.[5] A 2011 study sponsored by the same two groups plus the Association of periOperative Registered Nurses focused on nurses and nurse managers. Its findings were equally dismal:

- More than 80 percent of nurses expressed concerns about dangerous shortcuts, incompetence, and disrespect demonstrated by their colleagues.

- More than 50 percent said shortcuts led to near misses or harm; only 17 percent of this group had shared their concerns with colleagues.

- More than 33 percent said incompetence led to near misses or harm; and only 11 percent had spoken to the colleague considered incompetent.

- More than 50 percent said that disrespect prevented them from getting others to listen to them or respect their professional opinion; only 16 percent had confronted their disrespectful colleagues.[6]

In some ways, we might conclude, poor communication remains the biggest danger of all to patient safety.

Think about a very simple conversation, one we now recognize as crucial: asking a colleague in a clinical setting whether he or she has washed his or her hands prior to examining a patient. Stephen Evans, chairman of surgery at MedStar Georgetown University Hospital in Washington, DC, and a leader in patient safety, likes to pose this situation to medical students. You are in a room, he tells them, and the attending physician walks in and doesn't wash his hands. You say, "Excuse me, Dr. Evans. You forgot to wash your hands going into the room. Would you mind? I think it's important for patient safety."

Then, of course, comes the punch line: "What do you think happens?" Invariably there is nervous laughter among the doctors-in-training. Questioning superiors has not generally been part of the medical school curriculum. Hand washing is a simple thing, and by now every single clinician knows how important it is. But let me ask you, How many times have *you* witnessed somebody initiating that very simple yet very crucial conversation? It is hard. And most of us don't like "hard."

Health care systems are coming to understand the importance of crucial conversations. In November 2009, for instance, Advocate Health Care—the system of which Good Samaritan is a part—conducted a "leadership needs" assessment covering 1,500 managers across the entire system. Among the biggest needs identified were the ability to handle difficult conversations and the ability to manage conflict. In response, Advocate embarked on an enterprise-wide implementation of trainings in having crucial conversations. By January 2012 about 70 percent of the organization's leaders had completed the sixteen-hour program. Still, many systems remain in the Dark Ages when it comes to crucial conversations. One specialty hospital, for example, held its annual strategic planning retreat to discuss five organizational priorities. I had the honor of facilitating the retreat. Four of the five priorities were easy to discuss, because virtually everyone supported them. The fifth, succession planning, was highly important, because several top executives including the CEO were scheduled to retire in the next several years. Yet the group at the retreat voted to table this one—just as they had tabled it at several previous retreats.

Leaders of change teams cannot avoid hard conversations. If they are the kind of people who duck those difficult situations, the project is likely to fail. There are three reasons, all simple.

First, any project involves asking people to change—to do things differently, sometimes even to change their attitude. Nobody likes to change, so every project meets resistance. The conversations with the resisters are likely to be difficult.

Second, the project team itself may be contentious. Most teams in health care will contain at least a few individuals who believe that their training and experience qualify them to know nearly everything. Some teams will include people who have trouble getting along with others. Many will involve team members who are there under duress—and who just want to get things done as quickly as possible so they can get back to their "real" work. All of these situations are recipes for trouble, unless the project implementation leader and other team members are skilled at holding difficult conversations.

Third, most projects are likely to run into trouble in achieving their objectives. (If the goals were easy to attain, after all, there would be no need for an initiative.) At any given point, there is a risk of possible loss, defined both by the probability of loss and by the magnitude of loss if failure does occur.[7] The threat of failure looms larger as the expected value of the loss increases. When a project runs into trouble, the project implementation leader must confront the difficulty directly, preferably sooner rather than later, in three ways. He or she must report the situation to the project sponsor and perhaps the project and portfolio management review board. The project implementation leader must alert the project team and deal with people who may be contributing to the risk of failure. Finally, he or she must make whatever changes are necessary. All of these actions are likely to involve difficult—crucial—conversations. Delaying any of those conversations increases the risk of failure.

There is little mystery as to why crucial conversations are so hard. We human beings tend to hold things in. We fear the repercussions of expressing our views or feelings honestly and openly. We don't want to "drop a bomb" in a meeting, and we are uncomfortable when we seem to be attacking others or when we ourselves feel attacked. The trouble is, project work can't proceed successfully without these difficult conversations. *Making sure that they happen is the responsibility of the project implementation leader.* If you expect your projects to succeed, you will need a leader who can handle that responsibility.

EMOTIONAL INTELLIGENCE

"The rules for work are changing," wrote Goleman. "We're being judged by a new yardstick: not just by how smart we are, or by our training and experience, but also by how well we handle ourselves and each other."[8] Goleman is the psychologist and science writer who introduced the term *emotional intelligence (EI)* to the public in 1995 with his best-selling book *Emotional Intelligence: Why It Can Matter More Than IQ.*[9] Since then, he and many other people have written widely on the subject.

There are many different definitions of EI. Goleman has said it "refers to the capacity for recognizing our own feelings and those of others, for motivating ourselves, and for managing emotions in ourselves and in our relationships."[10] Two other EI specialists, Travis Bradberry and Jean Greaves, have refined it as "your ability to recognize and understand emotions in yourself and others, and your ability to use this awareness to manage your behavior and relationships."[11] Whatever anyone's exact wording may be, EI is a fundamentally intuitive concept. People with a high degree of EI understand their own emotions and are not at the mercy of them. They pick up on the emotions of others, and respond with sensitivity. They are empathic. Those with low EI, conversely, are like bulls in the social china shop, blundering their way through emotional situations that they do not fully understand. They lack empathy, and they lack insight into the role emotions play in social interaction. Psychologists have developed methods of measuring EI that allow it to be quantified, much like IQ. But nearly everyone has a gut-level sense of who is strong in EI and who is not. We say things like, "She really gets what's going on" or "He seems to sense the mood of the group" or "He was so sensitive in dealing with that difficult situation." We also say things like, "She got carried away by her emotions" or "He just ignored everybody's feelings."

Effective leadership seems to depend heavily on emotional intelligence. Some 90 percent of the difference between average and outstanding leaders has been linked to EI. A meta-analysis of 156 samples described in ninety-six separate papers found that intelligence explains only about 4 percent of the variance in who becomes a leader and who does not; much of the rest can doubtless be attributed to EI.[12] It's easy to understand why. Individuals with high EI have the ability to connect with people. They seem believable and trustworthy. It is said of President Bill Clinton that, in conversation, he had the ability to make someone feel that he or she was the only person Clinton cared about right at that moment. No wonder he was an effective leader.

Repeated analyses have also found that emotional intelligence has a paramount role in performance on the job—any type of job. High scores in the five areas of EI—self-awareness, self-regulation, self-motivation, empathy, and people skills—have more influence on job success than technical or professional training. In fact, EI may be more important to success than IQ and technical skills combined. According to Bradberry and Greaves, EI "is so critical to success that it accounts for 58% of performance in all types of jobs" and is "the single biggest predictor of performance in the workplace."[13]

In the context of a change initiative, high EI allows an individual to manage matrix conflict, such as the tension between the project manager and the functional manager. It also allows people to handle conflict within the team itself. Project teams naturally have many disputes, typically around such issues as schedules, project priorities, resources, technical options, administrative procedures, cost, and interpersonal differences.[14] Team members with low EI may be inclined to take these disputes personally and remain at loggerheads with one another. Team members with high EI are far more likely to understand one another's point of view, to work through disagreements, and thereby to reach appropriate solutions. According to one study, teams with high EI levels "felt greater psychological safety with each other, had lower levels of conflict, made decisions more collaboratively together, and experienced greater team learning."[15]

Does this mean you should give everybody an emotional intelligence test before assigning him or her to a project, and then select only the high scorers? Hardly. You might find yourself with even fewer candidates than usual. As Kathryn Faguy pointed out in her article "Emotional Intelligence in Health Care," research indicates "that EI varies among health care professionals just as it does in the population as a whole."[16] So you may not find a lot of high scorers among your staff. Still, EI is a critical soft skill. The more people you can find with higher rather than lower EI, the more likely it is that your initiative will succeed. A test of EI is probably less important than a gut feeling. You want the people on your change team—and the leaders of all your change teams—to be empathic, sensitive, and able to deal with their own emotions and those of others. High EI is a seemingly straightforward but important soft skill, and it is easily overlooked in the usual search for technical expertise.

TRUST

The last soft skill I want to examine in some detail is the ability to trust and to inspire trust.

Trust is in many ways the essential ingredient of effective health care. Obviously effective care requires skilled, knowledgeable professionals. It requires all the tools of the health care trade, from antibiotics to scalpels.

It requires ORs and ERs and MRIs and all the other sophisticated facilities and pieces of equipment that contribute to good care. But if you don't have trust, what are any of these worth? Many patients won't come in. Those who do enter the system won't cooperate with their clinicians. Imagine, as I wrote in a previous book, *The Trust Prescription for Healthcare*, that you are a surgery patient: "You have been stripped naked, stuck with needles, and hooked up to unfamiliar and often frightening machines. The people in charge are strangers, wear strange costumes—masks sometimes cover their faces—and have strange customs. They use words that you do not understand. Yet they are about to knock you unconscious and cut open your body. How important is it that you trust the hospital and the people who work there?"[17]

Patients don't care how much you know, goes the well-worn aphorism, until they know how much you care. They won't trust you until they know how much you care, either.

People build trust in one another over time. But it isn't just familiarity that breeds trust; on the contrary, as another maxim tells us, familiarity often breeds contempt. A common problem in health care settings is lack of trust, regardless of how long people have worked together, and not just between patients and their caregivers. Physicians don't trust nurses. Nurses don't trust the physicians. Nobody trusts administrators or their supposed partners, insurance companies and regulators. What are the chances that an institution with such distrust can deliver good care? And what are the chances that a change initiative's team in such a setting will actually function smoothly and achieve its objectives?

Yet trust can be built. There are four essential elements (figure 6.1). The first is a collection of traits that has much in common with emotional intelligence: warmth, empathy, and genuineness. These are aspects of people's affective domain, the feelings they experience and provoke in others. A person who respects the emotional well-being of others, who exhibits concern and compassion, is far more likely to be trusted than someone who is cold, distant, or unempathic.

A second element is integrity. Some people see integrity as essentially a synonym for trust, but that's not quite right. In an organizational

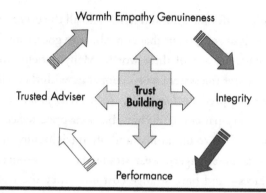

Figure 6.1 Four Domains of Trust Building

Source: Adapted from David A. Shore, *The Trust Crisis in Healthcare* (New York: Oxford University Press, 2007), 157–158.

context, integrity refers to how consistently an organization lives up to its promise—how frequently it acts fairly, justly, honestly, ethically. "If you have integrity, nothing else matters," said former senator Alan Simpson. "If you don't have integrity, nothing else matters." Human beings seem to have a hardwired ability to figure out who can be trusted and who cannot. An institution or a person without integrity will never be trusted, but one with integrity possesses a key building block of trust.

The third element is performance. I have emphasized in this book the importance of doing the right thing. But it is also important to do things right. Performance is how an individual or an organization follows through on its promise, on its business commitment. If the road to hell is paved with good intentions, so is the road to distrust. What counts in building trust, ultimately, is what people do and how they go about it, not what they say they will do.

The fourth element is a little different from the others. The first three were about creating trust. This one—the trusted adviser—is about a trusting *relationship*. If you are old enough, you will remember Walter Cronkite, the legendary CBS news anchor. For many years "Uncle Walter" was the most trusted man in America. People thought of him as a trusted adviser, unbiased and independent, a man who couldn't be bought. We often think of people in certain roles as trusted advisers. Nurses and pharmacists, for instance, are among the most trusted professionals in America. A good judge is regarded as an unbiased fact finder, trusted to deliver justice. A guidance counselor or coach may be a trusted mentor. And sometimes a person's nominal occupation makes no difference: we all know individuals whose advice we trust completely regardless of their job title. We feel comfortable consulting them. That feeling reflects the etymology of the word *trust*, which comes from the German word *trost*, meaning "comfort."

Trust exists when people's interactions with one another reflect and incorporate all four elements. In a change initiative, trust exists when everyone believes that the others on the team can be relied on, that they will act in the right way, and that they will do what they say. To really bring about change, a team must be united rather than divided. It must be a team with a shared vision. This will not occur in the absence of trust. Moreover, effective feedback is crucial to team performance. Without trust, there is no effective feedback, because people don't pay attention to or believe what others tell them.

• • •

This chapter has identified three critical soft skills that the people involved in change events need to have: the ability to hold crucial conversations, high emotional intelligence, and the ability to trust and inspire trust. Imagine an initiative that you have worked on. How would things have been different had the relevant people possessed these three skills? Now imagine one in which you may become involved. How important do you believe it is to find individuals with as much of these three skills as possible?

In my experience, it's essential. In the introduction to part 3 I discussed the apparent conflict between a "systems" approach and a "people" approach. In the end, however, it all comes down to people, if only because people create the systems. People also create change initiatives and are responsible for implementing them. When they can work collaboratively, with frank conversations and empathy and trust, change comes that much more easily.

SUMMARY

- Project teams need people with hard skills, such as clinical or technical abilities. But they also need people with soft skills.

- One essential soft skill is the ability to hold crucial conversations—to discuss difficult issues productively.

- A second is high emotional intelligence, meaning a sensitivity to others' emotions and one's own.

- A third is the ability to trust and engender trust.

NOTES

1. See the following page on the website of the Project Management Institute: http://www.pmi.org/en/Certification/Project-Management-Professional-PMP.aspx.
2. Project Management Institute, *Program Management 2010: A Study of Program Management in the U.S. Federal Government* (Newtown Square, PA: Project Management Institute, 2010), http://www.pmi.org/Business-Solutions/~/media/PDF/Business-Solutions/Government%20Program%20Management%20Study%20Report_FINAL.ashx.
3. Dave Zielinski, "Soft Skills, Hard Truths," *Training* 42, no.7 (2005): 18–22.
4. Adapted from Jeffrey K. Pinto, "Understanding the Role of Politics in Successful Project Management," *International Journal of Project Management* 18, no. 2 (2000): 85–91.
5. David Maxfield et al., *The Seven Crucial Conversations for Health Care* (Provo, UT: VitalSmarts, 2005).
6. David Maxfield et al., *The Silent Treatment: Why Safety Tools and Checklists Aren't Enough to Save Lives* (Provo, UT: VitalSmarts, 2011).
7. See Robert S. Billings, Thomas W. Milburn, and Mary Lou Schaalman, "A Model of Crisis Perception: A Theoretical and Empirical Analysis," *Administrative Science Quarterly* 25 (1980): 300–316.
8. Daniel Goleman, *Working with Emotional Intelligence* (New York: Bantam Books, 2000), 2.
9. Daniel Goleman, *Emotional Intelligence: Why It Can Matter More Than IQ*, 10th anniversary ed. (New York: Bantam Books, 2006).
10. Goleman, *Working with Emotional Intelligence*, 317
11. Travis Bradberry and Jean Greaves, *Emotional Intelligence 2.0* (San Diego, CA: TalentSmart, 2009), cited in Kathryn Faguy, "Emotional Intelligence in Health Care," *Radiologic Technology* 83, no. 3 (2012): 237–253.
12. Timothy A. Judge, Amy E. Colbert, and Remus Ilies, "Intelligence and Leadership: A Quantitative Review and Test of Theoretical Propositions," *Journal of Applied Psychology* 89 (2004): 542–552.
13. Bradberry and Greaves, *Emotional Intelligence 2.0*.
14. Rita Mulcahy, *Seven Sources of Project Conflict, in PMP Prep*, 7th ed. (Hopkins, MN: RMC, 2011).

15. Marcia Hughes and James Bradford Terrell, *The Emotionally Intelligent Team: Understanding and Developing the Behaviors of Success* (San Francisco: Jossey-Bass, 2007), cited in Faguy, "Emotional Intelligence in Health Care."
16. Faguy, "Emotional Intelligence in Health Care."
17. David A. Shore, *The Trust Prescription for Healthcare: Building Your Reputation with Consumers* (Chicago: Health Administration Press, 2005), xi.

7

Assembling the Individuals for a Change Event

Most companies have a well-developed system for assigning individual employees to change initiatives. They ask who is available. They look for people who have done something similar before, and people whom the responsible executive respects. Then they take whomever they can get. The result is that the same thirty people work on every project. As individuals, these people may be bright and talented, but often they participate only because they are willing and nobody else is. From an employee's perspective, the results of this catch-as-catch-can system are less than inspiring. Some folks seem always to be working on interesting projects. Others never get the chance to prove themselves. From the organization's perspective, relying on the same people every time is an all-around loss. Those frequent-project employees stretch themselves too thin. The talents and abilities of everyone else are never tapped.

As I hope to show here, you can do better. Not only can you identify people who possess the soft skills that will contribute to the success of a project, as described in chapter 6, but also you can identify the individual roles you need on each change team, and select people who are capable of filling those roles. You can ensure that no team grows too large, and that no individual has more project work than he or she can handle. You can create a project management human capital inventory, which should be capable of tracking both change leaders and potential team members. All these measures, to be discussed in this chapter, will help you find the right people and assign them to a project team. In chapter 8 I will take up the thorny issue of how to turn this disparate collection of individuals into a real team, one whose members can work together effectively and efficiently.

Let us look first at a question that many, many health care organizations never ask themselves at all: How many people does a project team require?

"DUNBAR'S NUMBER" FOR CHANGE TEAMS

We have sadly grown accustomed to horrific events in the headlines these days—bombings, mass shootings, and the like. But what happened to Kitty Genovese in 1964 was a different kind of tragedy. She was brutally stabbed to death in a quiet neighborhood in Queens, one of New York City's five boroughs. (I was a ten-year-old living in New York at the time.) Her killer attacked her in full view of neighboring apartment buildings; indeed, some thirty-eight people acknowledged hearing her screams and watching her being murdered. Yet no one—*no one*—called the police. When asked why, the typical response was, "I assumed someone else would call them." Later, two young social scientists began studying the behavior of bystanders, beginning with the Genovese stabbing. "Their startling conclusion," wrote *New York Times* columnist Joe Nocera not long ago, was "that the more people who witness a crime, the less likely any one of them will come to the aid of the victim."[1] This has become known as the *bystander effect*.

Most of us will recognize this phenomenon, which comes into play in everyday situations as well as in extreme ones. Some college students prefer large classes because there is less chance they will be called on to speak up (and therefore less need to keep up with the reading). Some employees, particularly in larger companies, duck responsibility for addressing an issue, figuring that someone else will worry about it. Some organizations fail to assign individual accountability, assuming that a whole department or group of people will take responsibility for a particular course of action. But when everyone is responsible, nobody is.

Many social scientists have studied the optimal size for groups of various sorts. The British anthropologist and Oxford University professor Robin Dunbar, for instance, has argued that the number of individuals with whom a person can maintain stable relationships is limited by the size of the human brain. "Dunbar's number," as it has come to be known, is around 150. (It is worth noting in light of this finding that Facebook limits any one person's number of "friends" to 5,000. I am not sure anybody really has 5,000 friends—or even 5,000 good acquaintances.) Dunbar's surveys seemed to approximate his predicted value, indicating 150 as the typical size of a Neolithic farming village, 150 as the splitting point for Hutterite settlements, and 150 as the basic unit size of professional armies in antiquity and in modern times since the sixteenth century.[2]

Is there a Dunbar's number—an ideal size—for change teams? Both theory and experience suggest that there is, and that it lies somewhere between seven and ten. My bias is toward seven, though with the caveat that if a typical project lasts nine months or a year, at least one member may have to drop off the team, and—as noted later on—it is good to have somebody on the bench. Of course, the actual number you arrive at will depend on the other considerations in this chapter, including getting the right mix of individuals who can play all the necessary roles.

The notion that seven is the ideal number for a change team may seem counterintuitive because so many teams in health care are considerably larger. But the research is compelling. Members' satisfaction with a group drops off sharply after seven, not peaking again until the group hits fifty (but that is a different kind of group). Once you have seven people in a group, some researchers argue, each additional member reduces the group's ability to make and execute decisions by about 10 percent.[3] People who have studied "lean" process improvement in factories and other settings have found that between six and nine members is the optimal team size.[4] In informal surveys of health care professionals who have attended my project management programs, I have found that the average team size in most organizations hovers around twelve—and that most participants believe that seven is the optimal size. Simply reducing the size accordingly would save about 40 percent of the cost in terms of project team members' time.

Why should a group's effectiveness decline as the group gets larger? One factor is surely the bystander effect: the bigger the group, the easier it is for any one individual to get by without contributing much, and when other members notice that one person is slacking off, they may be inclined to lower their own effort. A second factor: an increase in overhead costs. As groups get larger, they may spend more time discussing who should do what than they spend actually doing it. They must also spend more time addressing interpersonal issues, administrative matters, and so forth. The number of possible person-to-person links increases rapidly as the size of a group increases. A four-member group has six possible pairings, a twelve-member group sixty-six. Little wonder that larger groups find it hard to operate effectively. A useful heuristic for group size is what Intuit chief executive Brad Smith has called the two-pizza rule: if you can feed a team with two large pizzas, it isn't too big. If you need three pizzas, it probably is.

Small teams that undertake large initiatives do, of course, pose a risk: What happens if one or two members have to drop off the team? Organizations can mitigate this risk the same way juries do by having one or two alternate members. These individuals do not have to participate fully in the initiative. But they should be regularly informed of the project's discussions and progress, and they should expect to fill in if one of the current members has to depart. Bench strength is as valuable in projects as it is in a courtroom or on a playing field.

THE RIGHT MIXTURE OF PEOPLE

Chapter 6 discussed the soft skills that are desirable in every member of a change team, and particularly in the team leader: the ability to hold crucial conversations, high emotional intelligence, and the capacity to trust and to inspire trust. This chapter is about something different: assembling the right combination of skills in team members. After all, people differ in many ways. You want a team that is stronger than any of its individual members because it brings together people with complementary skills and attributes.

In part, this is a simple prescription: find people with the diverse technical skills required by the project. Most teams need to involve individuals from a variety of functions. You want representatives from every department or unit that will be deeply involved in the change, or whose participation is essential (IT, for instance). The exact composition will vary with the nature of the initiative. But the rest of the prescription is more complex and nuanced. You want different *kinds* of people, individuals who will contribute to the team in different ways.

Think, for example, about the phenomenon in basketball sometimes known as the "glue guy," the player who makes *everyone else* better. "There is a tension, peculiar to basketball, between the interests of the team and the interests of the individual," noted the journalist Michael Lewis. "The game continually tempts the people who play it to do things that are not in the interest of the group.... It is in basketball where the problems are most likely to be in the game—where the player, in his play, faces choices between maximizing his own perceived self-interest and winning. The choices are sufficiently complex that there is a fair chance he doesn't fully grasp that he is making them."

Lewis went on to discuss forward Shane Battier—then with the Houston Rockets, now with the Miami Heat—as the prototype of the glue guy, the individual who helps the team without racking up great statistics himself. He improves his teammates' rebounding. He may not shoot much, but he takes good shots and passes the ball to others who can do the same. Defensively, he guards a lot of the league's high scorers and reduces their shooting effectiveness. All in all, his teammates get better when he is on the court, and opponents get worse. "I call him Lego," Rockets general manager Daryl Morey told Lewis. "When he's on the court, all the pieces start to fit together. And everything that leads to winning that you can get to through intellect instead of innate ability, Shane excels in. I'll bet he's in the hundredth percentile of every category."[5]

Just as the stat sheets in basketball do not capture the true effect of a player's presence on the court (because they fail to take into account whether the player amassed shooting or rebounding statistics at the cost of hurting the team), so do many traditional metrics of team performance fail to capture the effect of the individual's chemistry on the group as a whole. People like Battier, who contribute indirectly by making other people better at what they do, are essential. As any athlete or computer scientist will tell you, approaches based on raw talent only take you so far. The mix of people on a team matters at least as much.

Another specific kind of mixture is equally important. I sometimes think of it as the "purple squirrel," a metaphor used by some human resources professionals to describe a job candidate with the ideal mix of hard and soft skills. But I have something slightly different in mind. Some people are naturally innovative, creative, imaginative, "right-brained" personalities. Others are naturally analytical, number-oriented, hard-nosed, "left-brained" personalities. Some of the most successful teams in business are combinations of these two types of personalities. At the Walt Disney Company, for instance, Walt was the creative visionary, the man who came up with the dreams, the chief "imagineer." His brother Roy Disney was the finance expert, the one who sold the dreams to bankers and suppliers. It was Roy who made the dreams come true. For instance, Walt's dream of a Disneyland-style park on the East Coast had moved only to the blueprint and early construction stage by the time he died in 1966. (While lying on his deathbed at Providence St. Joseph Medical Center, Walt had a map of the entire state of Florida projected onto the ceiling.) After Walt's passing, Roy came out of retirement to oversee the project. Walt Disney World opened in Lake Buena Vista (Orlando, Florida) in October 1971. Roy died two months later at age seventy-eight.[6] Walt and Roy together made a purple squirrel.

Writing in *Harvard Business Review*, Darrell Rigby and his coauthors, all Bain & Company consultants, called combinations such as the Disneys' "BothBrain" partnerships, noting that many other iconic duos fit this definition: Bill Hewlett and David Packard in technology (Hewlett-Packard), Hal Sperlich and Lee Iacocca in automobiles (first Ford and then Chrysler), Bill Bowerman and Phil Knight in sports equipment (Nike), and Howard Schultz and Orin Smith in food service (Starbucks).[7] In a business context, vision without execution is no more than daydreaming, and execution without vision is pointless busywork. These pairings avoid both pitfalls, which is why they are so powerful. Most project teams I have worked with would have benefited greatly from a little more vision or a little more focus on execution. Both are essential, which means that you need combinations of people with both kinds of skills—purple squirrels.

ROLES ON THE TEAM

So far I have discussed the traits or attributes you want to look for in change leaders and change team members. Now I want to widen the angle and look at what you need for the team itself. Just as a football team needs a quarterback, running backs, blockers, receivers, and so forth, a change team needs people to play specific roles (figure 7.1). But although every football coach knows his sport's lineup of positions, many health care organizations seem unaware that a change team should have an identified individual in every one of the necessary roles. We will now examine some of the core project stakeholders who are prominent early in the project life cycle.

Project Sponsor

Previous chapters described the role of the concept initiator and the project and portfolio management review board (PPMRB), so the first new role in figure 7.1 that bears mention here is that of the project sponsor.

This is one role that most organizations do understand: nearly every change initiative or project that I am familiar with has an executive sponsor. And every initiative or project needs a sponsor, badly. A project sponsor is an executive or higher-level manager who helps shepherd the project through all phases of its development, particularly the beginning

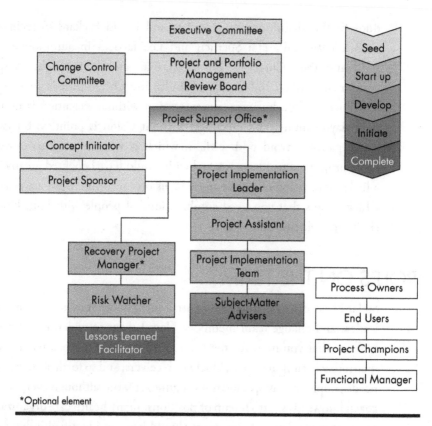

*Optional element

Figure 7.1 Core Project Stakeholders

stages. He or she may serve as an intermediary on behalf of the project to high-level executives, governing bodies, department heads, and any other entity beyond the reach of the project implementation leader. The project sponsor works with the project implementation team on issues of finance, judgment, project milestone status, and termination, and may present to the PPMRB. Most of the teams I have worked with have indicated that an engaged sponsor is a critical success factor, typically ranking it number one, two, or three among all factors. The problem is that large organizations often have hundreds of projects under way at any given time, yet have only a dozen or two dozen executives to act as sponsors. If each executive winds up with thirty or forty projects, he or she can't possibly engage with every one. Some executives have told me that they feel guilty because they cannot even list all the projects for which they are the sponsor, and because there are project teams on the list with whom they have never met.

The solution is simple: *sponsors* yes, *executives* not necessarily. Managers can be sponsors, particularly for smaller or less expensive projects. Directors will do nicely as sponsors for initiatives that are somewhat more complex or costly. Executive sponsorship should be reserved for the relatively few initiatives that are large, expensive, and critical to the organization's success. Table 7.1 shows one example of classifying projects: points are assigned to each category, and the sponsor is chosen accordingly. Other recommended components of a project sponsor classification might include the link to the strategic plan, the safety impact, and the level of risk. Determining sponsorship roles in this manner greatly expands an organization's capacity. It also provides professional growth and development opportunities for a wider range of managers while reducing the number of projects any one person is responsible for. And it increases the likelihood that projects will succeed.

It is critical, however, that each project have only one sponsor. That person takes ownership of the project and is accountable for its progress.

Table 7.1 Project Sponsor Classification

Project Class	Work Effort (Hours)	Staff Budget (Internal and External)	Sponsor Level
1	75–149	<$10,000	Manager
2	150–499	$10,000–24,999	Director
3	500–9,999	$25,000–499,999	Vice president
4	>10,000	>$500,000	Executive

If two or more people are listed as sponsors, each one is in danger of becoming a bystander, hoping that the other sponsor or sponsors will pick up the slack.

Project Implementation Leader (PIL)

Note the insertion of that word *implementation* into the conventionally defined role of project leader (also known as project manager). The project implementation leader is responsible for getting the initiative done. He or she remains for the duration of the project and is the single point of contact for anyone outside the team, the liaison through whom all communication must pass. If the PIL were a medical specialist, he or she would be a hospitalist—a physician who takes full responsibility for the care of a patient from admission through discharge. The PIL takes full responsibility for the initiative from beginning to end.

Who is the right individual? Project implementation leaders must know the industry, know the organization, and know the initiative at hand. They need superior team-building skills, including the ability to foster high performance and to facilitate robust, effective meetings. In smaller projects, the leader may be actively involved in doing project work. In larger ones, the leader manages the people who are actually performing the task. Leaders should be able to develop a *vision* of the project, usually working in conjunction with the concept initiator and the project sponsor; they should describe the *from* and the *to;* and they should be able to communicate why the status quo is inadequate and why the future state—the project's objectives—is preferable. They should make this vision relevant and understandable at every level of the organization, and they should be able to act as chief salesperson for the project's goals. Leaders need relevant technical skills, of course—but they also need the kinds of soft skills we have been discussing. Because they may have no formal authority whatsoever over team members, they need mental toughness, great negotiation skills, and the ability to inspire people to work toward a common end.

The precise job description of a PIL will vary with the nature of the project and of the organization itself. Most PILs will pick their team members, a key decision in any project, sometimes with the collaboration of the sponsor or the project management office (if there is one). Most will have full budget authority and the ability to commit the organization's resources up to a specified level. Whatever the level, the PIL oversees the deliverables for each stakeholder. He or she is the person accountable when something goes wrong, or when the initiative encounters unexpected bumps in the road.

As you can see, it is a difficult role. That is why good project managers in any setting are hard to find, and why the best command a high salary. Many health care organizations have been remiss in not seeking out individuals with the requisite skills, instead relying on what might be called "amateur" PILs. As is the case in any field, amateurs can sometimes turn in remarkable performances. Day in and day out, however, it is the professionals who do the better job.

"Leadership," according to James Kouzes and Barry Posner, "is the art of mobilizing others to want to struggle for shared aspirations."[8] A PIL needs to be able to exercise that kind of leadership—and if your initiative is led by such a person, you have greatly increased its chances of success.

Project Assistant

Many people in health care organizations have access to administrative support in their day job. Should we ask them to take on an additional task—work on a change team—*without* administrative support? It hardly seems reasonable.

The fact is, a talented project assistant is an invaluable aid to a change team. The assistant can schedule meetings, take attendance, update the charts, track down people who need to be contacted, and so on. The assistant can learn to use basic project management software, and help the PIL keep track of where things stand. He or she is a force multiplier, one who frees up the leader and team members for other work and thus improves overall efficiency. Not incidentally, assistants are paid considerably less than project managers—and may be better at administrative tasks. Tell potential PILs that they will be given a project assistant and they will be far more likely to say yes than if they believe they will have to handle all the administrative work themselves. Of course, one project assistant can support more than one project, depending on the size and complexity of each one.

Risk Watcher

One role listed in figure 7.1 is likely to be unfamiliar to nearly everybody: that of *risk watcher*. Just as the project and portfolio management review board needs one, so too does every change team that the board supervises. It is a critically important function.

Think about the initiatives you have worked on. In initiatives like these, the leader and (often) the sponsor may be on a mission to make their project successful. They are evangelists: they believe in the project, and they want everyone else to believe in it, too. Their team members engage in "happy talk," persuading one another that everything is going well and that there are no danger signs ahead. They do not want to hear about any risks, concerns, or potential trouble spots. Yet it is just this kind of thinking and behavior that lands so many initiatives in the soup. In effect, a team focused only on the positive is missing one of what the physician and author Edward de Bono called "six thinking hats." De Bono's taxonomy can be summarized like this:

White hat: information, facts

Yellow hat: benefits, value

Green hat: creativity, ideas

Red hat: feelings, intuition

Blue hat: managing the thinking process

The missing one—the black hat—focuses on cautions and concerns.[9] Wearing this hat is the job of the risk watcher.

Black-hat thinking is essential to any serious enterprise. It involves examining every issue from the point of view of what could go wrong.

It helps you spot fatal flaws and pitfalls before you embark on a course of action. It enables you to strengthen a plan's weak points. Of course, there are really two types of black-hat thinking. One involves a kind of Pareto analysis, often referred to as the 80:20 rule. In the case of risk it means that 80 percent of the risks are likely to stem from 20 percent of the inputs. Pareto analysis not only reveals the most important problems to solve but also provides a score showing the severity of the problem. A second kind of black-hat thinking is force-field analysis, which examines all the forces lined up on both sides of a plan, for and against. It helps you determine whether the plan is worthy of implementation—and if it is, where the biggest obstacles are likely to be found.

A risk watcher has a difficult job in that he or she must approach the task separately from the rest of the group. When everyone else is happy and enthusiastic, the risk watcher has to hold back, anticipate problems, and alert people to risks. The risk watcher is really a hedge against the well-known and often destructive phenomenon of groupthink. If, as artificial-heart pioneer Robert Jarvik once said, leaders are "visionaries with a poorly developed sense of fear and no concept of the odds against them," risk watchers are people who welcome fear and focus precisely on the odds against a project's success so as to improve them.

Project Implementation Team and Subject Matter Advisers

This notion needs no more than a word of explanation. Many health care organizations seem to believe that a change team must include experts in every relevant area. That makes the team large and unwieldy. Far better to keep core team membership in the vicinity of seven or eight, and to draw on designated subject matter advisers for expertise that goes beyond what the team itself possesses. When you hire a contractor to remodel your house, he or she is likely to have a core staff of skilled workers to handle most of the job. But he or she is also likely to contract out plumbing, electrical work, stonemasonry, and other specialties to experts in those fields. So it should be with change teams.

Project Champions

One other short note, on project champions. Project champions are cheer-leaders. They have no direct responsibility for project work or oversight; they are people who know of the initiative and think it will be good for their department or the entire organization. They talk it up. They can be relied on for support. They may provide a venue for pilots or other experiments, and they can be counted on to bring along others who are not so keen on change. The more champions an initiative has, the better. This means that the PIL and team members would do well to network and spread the word among friends and colleagues, in hopes of developing more and more champions.

THE RIGHT NUMBER OF PROJECTS

The analogue to a Dunbar's number for the size of a change team is a kind of Dunbar's number for the number of initiatives in an organization. How many projects can one organization support at any given time? This is essentially a question of organizational capacity or bandwidth. Most health care organizations undertake many, many projects. According to a 2010 survey, nearly half were involved in more than fifty, including about a quarter that were engaged in more than one hundred.[10] That most organizations regularly exceed their capacity should be evident from the fact that so many initiatives wind up lost in the woods, never succeeding and never really failing, each one just another venture that didn't quite turn out as people had hoped. If an organization undertakes too few initiatives, however, it is likely to miss some opportunities and fall behind its competitors.

There are at least three limits on an organization's bandwidth. One is the availability of money and time. A second is the availability of executives, managers, or others to oversee and take responsibility for projects. A third is the availability of project implementation leaders and people to work on project teams. It is often tempting for senior administrators to "load up" sponsors, leaders, and team members with three or four projects or more. But it is risky. As the number of projects people work on increases, the effectiveness of those individuals is likely to decline. Anyone who has contributed to many projects at once knows that there are significant switching costs, just because you must frequently reorient yourself and catch up with a new set of facts.

So how many initiatives should be undertaken at once? Some organizations draw a bright line under the number of change initiatives they will launch each year (for example, Thedacare, the Wisconsin network of medical centers, undertakes only five). Others vary the number from year to year, relying on historical data to determine their current capacity to deliver on initiatives. This method, of course, is only as good as the availability and quality of the data. Still others rely on benchmarking, looking at other organizations that are similar to see what the industry standard is.

The answer, therefore, is undoubtedly "it depends." But guidelines may be helpful. Add up the number of project implementation leaders you have available. If your initiatives are small or medium size, each leader may be able to manage more than one. So twelve PILs, for instance, might be able to take on eighteen not-too-big projects. For your organization, count the number of potential sponsors and multiply that by the number of projects each one can be responsible for. If you have nine potential sponsors and each can handle two projects, that is eighteen. Finally, allow for unplanned or mandated projects that may crop up in the course of a year. If that number is three, then your organizational capacity in terms of human resources is eighteen minus three, or fifteen. You will need to perform similar calculations to ensure that the budgetary resources are there as well. Add up the budgets for all projects, and be sure that the total does not exceed the organization's overall budget for projects.

These are just simple calculations, of course. They are complicated, however, by the commonly used federated model in health care, in which departments and sites have a high degree of autonomy. Some projects will be centralized, others decentralized, and it may be difficult to coordinate the necessary estimates. Still, having any estimate of an organization's bandwidth is better than flying blind.

THE PROJECT MANAGEMENT HUMAN CAPITAL INVENTORY

We live in an age of networks and databases. Match.com, to take just one example, allows people looking for romantic partners to search by height, body type, education, faith, ethnicity, and many other variables (including, curiously, marital status). Suppose a project implementation leader were able to search a database of potential team members that showed a host of relevant variables. These might include education and training; experience; personality profile (Myers-Briggs Type Indicator, for example); current project activities (so the leader could assess an individual's availability); complementary assets, such as additional skills or talents; and perhaps a snapshot of the performance level of the operating group from which a person might be drawn. Such a database would make possible a quick initial screening of people to interview, and it would help an organization balance its resources, so that the choice of individuals to serve on a project team not only would make a good team but also wouldn't leave regular operations in the lurch. Organizations too often focus on securing a budget, IT resources, and other necessary elements when they consider launching a project. They forget until the last minute about the people who must be involved. Creating a project management human capital inventory would remind everyone that people come first, and that it need not be an impossible chore to select the right ones.

DO PEOPLE MAKE A TEAM?

This chapter has gone into some detail on the factors and methods that are relevant to selecting people for a project team. I do not mean to burden you with a dozen different sets of guidelines and checklists and recommendations. But few decisions in a project launch are as important as those relating to personnel. The right leader, and the right combination of team members, can make all the difference in regard to success and failure. It is worth spending extra time and effort at the front end, so that you do not have to spend too much time cleaning up messes at the back end.

There is one more job we have to examine: taking those individuals you have selected and making them into an effective, efficient project team. That is the subject of chapter 8.

SUMMARY

- Project teams shouldn't be too big. The "Dunbar's number" for optimal team size is probably about seven.

- Project teams need people with diverse sets of skills, both left-brained analytical types and right-brained creative types.

- Every team needs individuals in defined roles, including project implementation leader, project assistant, and risk watcher. Teams can be supported by subject matter advisers, project sponsors, and project champions.

- An organization should take on only as many projects as it can support. A project management human capital inventory will enable the organization to deploy people with the right project experience, and will prevent these individuals from being assigned to too many projects.

NOTES

1. Joe Nocera, "It's Hard to Be a Hero," *New York Times*, December 7, 2012.
2. Robin Dunbar, *How Many Friends Does One Person Need? Dunbar's Number and Other Evolutionary Quirks* (Cambridge, MA: Harvard University Press, 2010).
3. Marcia W. Blenko, Michael C. Mankins, and Paul Rogers, *Decide and Deliver: Five Steps to Breakthrough Performance in Your Organization* (Boston: Harvard Business School Press, 2010), 133.
4. George Koenigsaecker, *Leading the Lean Enterprise Transformation* (New York: CRC Press), 66–68.
5. Michael Lewis, "The No-Stats All Star," *New York Times Magazine*, February 13, 2009.
6. See Bob Thomas, *Walt Disney: An American Original* (New York: Hyperion Books, 1976).
7. Darrell K. Rigby, Kara Gruver, and James Allen, "Innovation in Turbulent Times," *Harvard Business Review* 86, no. 6 (June 2009): 79–86.
8. James Kouzes and Barry Posner, *The Leadership Challenge*, 5th ed. (San Francisco: Jossey-Bass, 2012).
9. Edward de Bono, *Six Thinking Hats* (New York: Back Bay Books, 1999).
10. *Project Portfolio Management and Project Management Trends in Healthcare Survey Results* (Newtown, PA: PMI Healthcare SIG, February 2010).

8

Converting Individuals into a Project Implementation Team

Let us imagine that you have selected the right initiative, one that is consistent with your organization's mission, vision, and values (MV^2) and that promises to further its strategic goals. You have also chosen the right people to serve on the change team. It is a group of seven or eight. It does not rely on all the usual suspects. It does include individuals with the diverse mix of skills, personality types, and roles discussed in chapter 7. Now there is only one problem. You do not have a change team, you have a bunch of folks who may never have worked together and who have only a rudimentary idea of what they are there for and what they are supposed to do. This is when the project implementation leader (PIL) must forge the group into a real team. It begins with the process known as *onboarding*.

ONBOARDING A GROUP

The term *onboarding* is typically reserved for the orientation and acclimation period most companies provide for new hires, and for all the HR-sponsored activities that take place during that period. There is the obligatory tour of the office or facilities. There are the training sessions, often complete with get-to-know-you games. There is the address by the CEO or the senior vice president in charge of the unit. At some organizations, onboarding in one form or another can last for a week or more. Others limit it to half a day at most.

But when it is done right, onboarding works. According to one study, 84 percent of best-in-class organizations included formal training programs for new hires in the onboarding process, and new employees who participated in these programs achieved optimal levels of productivity faster than others did.[1] In another study, effective onboarding was found to improve employee performance by more than 11 percent.[2] Texas Instruments found that employees who go through onboarding reach full productivity levels at least two months earlier than did others.[3]

Onboarding for a change team is just as important as onboarding for an organization, but it is a little different. There are no accepted rituals or protocols and no HR staff to lead the process. There is no preexisting group into which one or two new individuals must now fit. There is only a task at hand: *take this group of disparate people from all over the organization and get them focused on the same task and working together collaboratively*. That can be particularly trying when, as is often the case, project team members come from different locations and must sometimes collaborate virtually. The less face time people have with one another, the more likely it is that the team and the project will seem like something apart, something "other," not an essential element of any individual's daily responsibilities.

Achieving this task of melding group members is essential to success. Without it, initiatives will begin to dissipate. You will find that meetings are starting late and ending later, that they are hamstrung by private agendas or personal disputes, that team members are multitasking when they should be focusing on the job at hand. You will find that members are disengaged from the project, and that communication is inefficient. The team will begin to miss its deadlines, and morale will suffer. It will be spending thousands of dollars of the organization's money on lost time and wasted effort.

BEGINNING THE ONBOARDING PROCESS: DAY ZERO

The primary purpose of onboarding in this context is to create enthusiastic and dedicated team members who not only can work effectively together but also feel a sense of ownership of the project. Behavioral economists call it the "endowment effect": the fact that nearly all of us tend to value things more once we feel that we own those things. And it doesn't matter what the "thing" is—it can be a car, a house, a job, or a trivial object, such as a coffee mug. Team members value the initiative more as they come to feel that it is theirs. They will feel responsibility for the project's outcomes, which is an indispensable precondition for success.

How does a team develop that sense of ownership? It starts even before the group's first meeting—on what I like to call day zero. Just as wise employers get new hires involved even before their first day of work, a wise project implementation leader will begin to involve team members as soon as they are selected and accept the appointment. The leader gives each member a note of welcome from the initiative's sponsor, which spells out the importance of the initiative to the organization's strategic vision. It is essential to keep that big picture front and center in everyone's mind. The leader also gives people his or her own welcome, perhaps describing the background of the project. The leader provides profiles of him- or herself and of the other team members, so that all will know a little something about their new colleagues.

Day zero also includes distributing the plan of concept. This should be required reading for everyone, and it should include the project and portfolio management review board's scoring of the project and accompanying commentary. Now members begin to see that what they are working on *matters*—that people elsewhere in the organization are taking it seriously, and are counting on the team to bring it to fruition. The leader also ensures that new team members have access to all the background information regarding the initiative that is available on the organization's intranet. He or she then begins discussions with each team member about the initiative's objectives, and asks them if there is any additional information they can provide that would be helpful. The goal is to ensure that each person feels like a valuable member of this still-forming group, and that everyone has relevant information on the scope and goals of the project. All of these measures begin to establish a positive trajectory. They encourage team members to hit the ground running when the project commences.

THE NEXT STEP: DAY ONE

Soon after the day zero preparations are complete comes day one, the first meeting.

This is a critical point in an initiative's life. Some people will be getting to know each other for the first time. Many will be forming their first impression of the PIL as a leader. A few team members will be nervous; some will be skeptical; many will be trying to make a favorable first impression. Two things can help this meeting get off to a good start. First, make it a celebratory kickoff, not just an introductory gathering. Invite people from senior management to meet the group, to describe the importance of the initiative, and to lend their support. Offer lunch or cake or some other added attraction. Provide team members with a small welcome gift. You are asking them to put in discretionary effort to help the organization on some essential task. Make sure you communicate that the organization values the extra effort.

Second, have every essential item ready to go when team members walk in. Printed agendas. Packets of information. Name tags. A whiteboard or some other method of sharing input and communication. Here, too, you want to convey some unspoken messages. *This is a serious project, and we are approaching it in a businesslike manner. It is not just a little something that we are doing on the side, whenever we might feel like it.*

The meeting has several tasks in addition to making people feel welcome and helping them get to know one another. It should outline and emphasize the project's goals and strategic importance. It should define short-term and long-term priorities. It should lay out short-term and middle-term assignments. I am not suggesting that the PIL simply issue orders. He or she must take the lead, but the meeting will be much more productive if everyone gets a chance to offer input, discuss the topics, and then volunteer for tasks.

The leader will also need to define the working relationships he or she expects as the group goes about its tasks. These specifications include the frequency and methods of communication among members; the levels of administrative or technical support that will be made available to the team; and the extent of organizational or outside resources that they can count on. The leader should determine what each team member needs from the organization and from him or her to succeed in the assigned tasks. The group should discuss the challenges or obstacles that might get in the way. The group also should reach consensus on a "terms of engagement" agreement, establishing team-wide expectations. The point here is to help team members feel productive *as part of the group* right from the start. Tackling real problems together helps everyone get past that initial nervousness or skepticism; it begins to create a team where before there were only individuals.

One other idea is important to introduce in this meeting: the "general theory of second best." Most change initiatives begin with a set of objectives. But the list of objectives quickly grows. You have probably been part of such a process. Someone says, "As long as we are doing X, we should really also do Y." Another person chimes in, "And Z would make the situation even better." The number of nice-to-haves can quickly spiral out of control, particularly because many people will be new to the task at hand. It is up to the project implementation leader to rein in this tendency and keep people focused on the original list of objectives, reducing the likelihood of scope creep. The ideal solution is rarely the best one—it is likely to be too costly, to take too much time, or even to be impossible to achieve. "Second best"—what can be accomplished in the real world, in a reasonable amount of time, at a reasonable cost—is what the change team should seek. It is better to have accomplished 80 percent of the ideal than to fail at achieving 100 percent.

When the initial meeting has moved from the welcoming and the introductions to the business at hand, it should be run just as future team meetings will be run. The group should stick to its agenda and to each item's allotted time. The objective should always be dialogue among members, not unfocused discussion or debate. What's the difference? Dialogue is based on equality, camaraderie, an absence of coercive influences. People listen to one another with empathy; they take each other's points of view seriously. They bring assumptions out into the open. They don't try to score points; they do try to find common ground. When the discussion begins to stray, it is the leader's job to refocus it on the topic at hand.

At the end of the meeting, the group should review and evaluate what it accomplished. Group members should ask, "Did we get through our agenda items? Did we document actions, results, and ideas? Did we recognize everyone's contributions and celebrate our achievements?" Action-oriented minutes can be extremely helpful in this context as day one moves on to day two and all the days thereafter. The minutes should spell out not only what was discussed but also what was decided, and who is responsible for follow-up action. That makes it easy to check back at the following weekly meeting and ensure that all the tasks were done.

DECISIONS AND TRACKING

Every group, from the officers aboard an aircraft carrier to a parent-teacher association, has to know how it will make decisions. The spectrum ranges from *directive*—decisions are made by one individual, no questions asked—to *consensus*, whereby decisions must be agreed to by every member of the group. In between are *democratic* forms of decision making, usually one vote per person, and *participative* forms, in which one person makes the decision after consultation with others.

Which form of decision making should the project team adopt? Some organizations expect every unit and group to operate according to similar principles. If that is the case, then the only task at the first meeting is to remind everyone of the organization's preferred form and explain how it works. Most organizations, however, leave the decision to individual groups or team leaders. "Deciding how to decide" is a critically important step. In some cases, groups will function democratically or by consensus. In others, the leader may feel that he or she must make the ultimate decisions. If that is the case, the leader has a responsibility to spell out how, and to what extent, he or she will consult with others. For instance, the leader may ask the group (or a few individuals) to recommend a course of action, with the understanding that he or she will make the final choice. The leader may ask others in the organization for input, and may give veto power to people inside or outside of the group if the decision at hand cannot go forward without those individuals' approval.

Whatever the decision-making practice, remember that effective execution of a decision is every bit as important as the decision itself. "We like to give audiences a quiz about three frogs on a log," wrote three experts on decision making in organizations. "One frog decides to jump off; how many are left on the log? Though they know it's a trick question, listeners are often baffled. Some say two, the obvious choice; others say zero, figuring the first frog rocked the log and knocked the others off. But the real answer is three, because deciding to do something isn't the same as doing it. This homely lesson applies doubly to [a] change effort: if you don't take action, the whole thing will peter out."[4]

That is why I suggest reviewing decisions at the end of every meeting, just to make sure that everyone understands what was decided and who is responsible for executing the decision.

There are many good books available on tracking the schedule and budget of a project, so I will not go into any depth on this subject. Suffice it to say that one task that should be accomplished in each meeting is to compare the original schedule to the schedule to date, using whatever form of tracking tool makes sense for this particular initiative. It is the same for the budget: projected expenditures need to be compared to actual expenditures, so that the team knows whether it is on course financially. If either the schedule or the financials are significantly off course, the team will want to take corrective action. The action-oriented minutes should reflect this. (For example, "The schedule slippage for task 13 will be resolved by assigning additional resources from the temporary pool. Richard agreed to be responsible for managing the catch-up.")

At a minimum, onboarding should accomplish three tasks. Every team member should have a good understanding of the project—that is, what it is, what it hopes to accomplish, and how long it is likely to take. Every member should understand his or her role, and every member should know the project's key performance indicators. Between-meeting activities should reinforce these understandings. The leader or the project assistant can regularly update the intranet, posting meeting write-ups, schedules, and relevant materials. The leader can continue to clarify the team's mandate, objectives, and performance measures should there be any confusion. Communication among team members should not be limited to meetings; on the contrary, the leader in particular needs to be in regular touch with members, getting feedback on their progress in accomplishing specific tasks. The leader can also gather feedback on the team itself, on the project, and on team meetings, thereby encouraging continuous improvement.

PASSION AND ENTHUSIASM

Notice I started the previous paragraph with "at a minimum." That paragraph outlined the left-brained, rational, task-oriented part of a team, which is essential. But there is another aspect of every team: the emotional side. It addresses the issue of how much team members *care* about whether the initiative succeeds. I think of it as the "gung ho onboarding continuum" (figure 8.1).

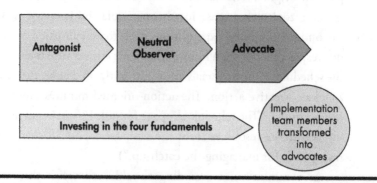

Figure 8.1   Gung Ho Onboarding Continuum

Look at the figure. The four fundamentals are alignment, passion, engagement, and trust. On the left are "antagonist" and "neutral observer." When the project begins, most team members are likely to be relatively neutral on the idea, just because they do not know a lot about it. A few may be skeptics. Over time, the PIL and the team itself should turn more and more team members into enthusiastic advocates—gung ho participants. A team, after all, is not simply a group of people; it is a group of people who are coordinated and united, fixed on achieving the same goal, and animated by a collective spirit of enthusiasm. Think of a sports team. Winners execute better, to be sure. But they do so, usually, because they are fired up about beating their opponents. As Sun Tzu put it in *The Art of War*, "He will win whose army is animated by the same spirit throughout its ranks."[5] Change teams aren't trying to vanquish an opponent—except maybe the status quo—and they certainly are not an army. But they will achieve their goals more effectively, and have more fun in the process, if they feel passionate about the task at hand. Passion leads to commitment and to discretionary effort. With passion, virtually everything becomes possible. Without passion, project work degenerates into drudgery.

Where do passion and enthusiasm come from? With change initiatives, they start at the beginning, with the concept initiator. The concept initiator is bound to be passionate about the project, just because it was his or her idea. The initiator cared enough about it to write it up, discuss it with others, refine it, and submit it to the project and portfolio management review board. The board was presumably enthusiastic about the project; otherwise board members would not have approved it. (If an initiative does *not* generate passion among board members, forget it.) The project implementation leader should be passionate—and should convey that passion to team members from the very first. "This initiative matters. This will make a big difference to our organization, to our patients and colleagues, and to our own work lives." The PIL has to transfer information, of course, but unless he or she also transfers enthusiasm, the project launch will not be successful. After all, most people in an organization do not want to change. Unless people are passionate about change—unless they can convey their excitement and enthusiasm about a better future state—inertia will win the day. Robert Kraft, owner of the New England Patriots football team, once said, "If you're passionate about winning and you help put an organization in place that can win, the business part will follow."[6] If members of the change team are not passionate about the goal at hand, they should resign from the assignment. The famous dancer and choreographer Martha Graham once said, "Great dancers are not great because of their technique; they are great because of their passion."[7] What makes a change team great is its passion to reach the project's objectives.

ALIGNMENT

Walt Disney once said, "Of all the things I've done, the most vital is coordinating those who work with me and aiming their efforts at a certain goal."[8] If you doubt the importance of alignment, check out the famous Monty Python skit "The 100-Yard Dash for People with No Sense of Direction," available on YouTube. At the gun, of course, all the runners race off in different directions. It's funny when Monty Python does it, but it is not funny when project team members begin working at cross-purposes, or simply without any sense of coordination.

When we picture something we want to create—and that is essentially what a project team must do—what we really do is imagine a vision of the future, which also makes plain the difference between that future state and the current one. Every creative artist understands this principle; Robert Fritz called it "structural tension."[9] A change team wants to bridge its structural tension so that everyone shares the same vision. It may help if team leaders regularly offer a reality check: "This is the direction in which we are headed; this is our goal; here is what we have done so far to move toward our goal." When people bring up a vision that is not shared, they can be gently guided back onto the common path.

Ascension Health is a large Catholic health care system in the United States, with more than five hundred locations in twenty states and the District of Columbia. It is also one of the nation's most respected systems, partly because it has focused extensively on measures to increase patient satisfaction. In 2008 the system published its "five principles of activating change." The first was, "Commission an inspired and inspirational affinity group to lead the charge." The second was, "Develop and communicate a clear, workable goal." To me, these are essentially synonyms for passion and alignment, respectively.

TRUST

I want to close out this chapter with one more short discussion of trust, because if you don't have high levels of trust, then every change initiative you launch is likely to fail. And building trust is an essential element of converting an assemblage of individuals into an effective change team.

I have written extensively about trust in the larger context of health care. (See, for example, *The Trust Prescription for Healthcare*.[10]) In this book we have already discussed the ability to trust and to engender trust as a requisite soft skill for team leaders and members (chapter 6). Here I want to review just a few main points in the context of this chapter, because trust is indispensable to the enterprise of change. The organization must trust the team to accomplish its goals. The leader must trust individual team members to do their part. Individual members must trust that the organization and the leader will support them and provide them with the necessary resources. They must also trust one another: they must believe that all the members will do what they say they will do, that they will be straight with each other, and that there will be no hidden agendas. Note that when I say "trust" I do not mean "hope and pray." Every organization must track its progress toward agreed-on goals, and change teams are no exception. But "trust and track" is a very different style of operation from the traditional management method of "command and control," which is explicitly based on an absence of trust.

Confucius told his disciple Tsze-kung that every government needs three things: weapons, food, and trust. If a ruler cannot maintain all three, the great teacher added, he should give up weapons first and food next. Trust should be guarded to the end, because "without trust we cannot stand."

Health care organizations need their weapons, of course: they need drugs, diagnostic instruments, and medical devices of all sorts. They need food, which I take as a metaphor in this context for patient care. And they need trust. Trust mediates therapeutic processes. It has an indirect influence on health outcomes through its impact on patient satisfaction, adherence to treatment regimens, and continuity with a provider. Higher levels of trust encourage patients to seek out health care and disclose appropriate information, thus making accurate and timely diagnoses possible.[11] When trust fails—and unfortunately it too often does—the result is disenrollment in health care programs, more demands for referrals, increased litigation, poorer adherence to recommended treatments, more weight placed on negative events, lower participation in clinical trials, and lower participation in organ donation. It is hard to see how any health care system can effectively function without high levels of trust.

Trust is equally important in the employer-employee relationship, and there, too, it is often lacking. Only 39 percent of employees at U.S. companies say they trust the company's senior leaders. Only one-third of employees believe that employers do business with honesty and integrity. This is a sad situation, because, according to the research organization Great Place to Work, employee trust levels and corporate performance are closely connected. Great Place to Work surveys have also regularly found that trust is the single most important element encouraging employees to commit to an organization.[12] Without trust, the organization has said, people operate as individuals rather than as fully participating members of the same team; groups operate as "functional islands"; and the organization as a whole suffers. By contrast, in a workplace with high levels of trust, many good things happen. Individuals become more innovative—a requirement for success in any business these days, but especially in health care. Teams collaborate more effectively, and employees are more likely to feel engaged in their work. Little wonder that corporate performance tends to improve.[13] For example, companies named the "100 Best Companies to Work For in America" obtained 2.3 to 3.8 percent better annual stock returns than comparable companies between 1984 and 2011.[14]

It is not hard to understand why trust is so important. In a society, trust enables people to do business with one another without undue reliance on contracts, laws, regulations, police supervision, and so forth. High-trust societies have regularly been found to be more productive than low-trust societies. In health care, trust enables patients to submit to the peculiar customs and rituals of what is, after all, an alien world—the doctor's office or the medical center or the hospital. (Would you let just anybody give you something to swallow, or inject you with a needle?) In the workplace, trust enables people to work together without internal contracts, written agreements, or close management supervision. Work is therefore far more productive than it otherwise would be, because people are not spending time policing each other. Trust also enables people to take risks—to try new things, to work with new people, to conduct new experiments. This is why it encourages innovation.

People who work on a change team have embarked on a journey. They have an objective in mind that is by definition new and thus uncertain. They are taking risks—devoting time and resources to efforts that may fail or backfire in unpredictable ways. They cannot reach their objectives unless they can work together fruitfully. How can any of this happen without high levels of trust? As onboarding proceeds, as teams build enthusiasm and passion and alignment, remember to take the group's "trust temperature" regularly. If people do not trust one another, everything else you do will be for naught.

SUMMARY

- Onboarding—with prescribed activities for "day zero" and day one—can help forge a team out of a disparate group of individuals.

- A key part of the process is for the team to agree on how it will make decisions.

- A team leader needs to generate passion and enthusiasm among the group, and align it around the project's objectives.

- A high level of trust within the project team is a critical success factor. Building trust is an essential part of the leader's job.

NOTES

1. Aberdeen Group, *All Aboard: Effective Onboarding Strategies and Techniques* (Boston, MA: Aberdeen Group, 2007), http://www.aberdeen.com/Aberdeen-Library/4617/RP-effective-onboarding-strats.aspx.
2. Corporate Executive Board, *Recruiting Roundtable Survey 2005* (Arlington, VA: Corporate Executive Board, 2005).
3. Rebecca Ganzel, "Putting Out the Welcome Mat," *Training* 35, no. 3 (1998), 54.
4. Marcia W. Blenko, Michael C. Mankins, and Paul Rogers, *Decide and Deliver: 5 Steps to Breakthrough Performance in Your Organization* (Boston: Harvard Business Review Press, 2010), 133.
5. Sun Tzu, *The Art of War* (1910; repr., London: Pax Librorum, 2009), 11.
6. Quoted in Scott Rosner and Kenneth Shropshire, *The Business of Sports* (Sudbury, MA: Jones & Bartlett, 2011), 14.
7. Quoted in Kevin Nelson, *The Runner's Book of Daily Inspiration: A Year of Motivation, Revelation, and Instruction* (New York: McGraw-Hill, 1999), 11.
8. Quoted in R. Lynn Wilson, *Exploring Great Leadership: A Practical Look from the Inside* (Bloomington, IN: iUniverse, 2012), 86.
9. Robert Fritz, *Creating* (New York: Fawcett, 1991).
10. David A. Shore, *The Trust Prescription for Healthcare: Building Your Reputation with Consumers* (Chicago: Health Administration Press, 2005).
11. See, for example, Michael Calnan and Rosemary Rowe, *Trust in Health Care: An Agenda for Future Research* (London: Nuffield Trust, 2004).
12. "What Are the Benefits?" Great Place to Work, accessed May 6, 2013, http://www.greatplacetowork.com/our-approach/what-are-the-benefits-great-workplaces.
13. See http://www.greatplacetowork.com.
14. Alex Edmans, "The Link between Job Satisfaction and Firm Value, with Implications for Corporate Social Responsibility," *Academy of Management Perspectives* 26 (November 2012): 1–19.

9

The First Mile and Beyond

Like most people, I am convinced that the health care system needs change—certainly in the United States, but probably all around the world as well. The introduction to part 1 of this book outlined some of the reasons. Yet it hardly matters what you or I think about the necessity of change. Advocate it or not, welcome it or not, change is happening every day. Governments and other stakeholders continually place new obligations and new restrictions on health care organizations. Sometimes they offer those organizations new opportunities as well. Consumers come with new expectations. Health care technologies continue to evolve. Standing still in the midst of this maelstrom is not an option for anybody.

There can be no change without change events. Call them initiatives, call them projects, call them whatever you like—they are the key to reshaping how health care organizations go about their business. Absent purposeful intervention, any organization will always do tomorrow pretty much what it did today. Organizations require a deliberate move, a project, if they are to do things differently. It is therefore safe to conclude that the current haphazard proliferation of projects in nearly every health care setting will continue, and indeed will get worse. Peter Drucker once said that the modern era is the age of the knowledge worker. In health care, we can say that it is the age of the project worker. You cannot pursue a career in this field without expecting to contribute at some point to change initiatives. And you cannot run an organization without learning to launch and manage change initiatives effectively.

All this change is stressful, both for organizations and for the individuals who staff them. People often fear change. They don't want to trade a situation they know for one they don't know. And most organizations don't have a good system for launching change events, instead relying on what might be called the French Foreign Legion model: pat people on the rump and send them out into the desert. To be sure, there are good ideas for change all over the place, many of them bubbling up from rank-and-file employees. But what counts most, ultimately, is the ability to execute. There is a big gap between ideas and implementation, just as there is between basic biomedical research and the emergence of new treatments for patients. To change successfully, health care organizations don't need *reflexive* actions, autonomic responses to a stimuli. Rather, they need *reflective* actions, plans of action based on thought and deliberate intent. "Just Do It" works fine as a slogan for athletes, but it is not a recipe for successful projects.

My argument in this book is that the key determinants of project success—the factors that will let you bridge that gap between ideas and implementation—lie mainly in the first mile.

Albert Einstein purportedly (and possibly apocryphally) said that if he had twenty days to solve a problem, he would spend nineteen days defining it. So it is with change events. If you can get all the first steps right, if you can answer the *why* as well as the *what*, the *how*, the *when*, and the *who*, you will be well on your way to a successful project. The middle and final miles are important, to be sure. (The middle mile in particular is the stuff of conventional project management texts, and you will need the kind of expertise those books describe and impart.) But if you don't get off to a good start, no amount of project management expertise will enable your initiative to succeed. It will crash and burn before it ever reaches cruising altitude.

Let us review what the first mile entails.

Right from the start, it involves adopting a different mind-set about change (chapter 1). Our thoughts, attitudes, and assumptions govern how we approach a problem. If you can accept the necessity and the inevitability of change, if you can adopt the mind-sets of marketers and manufacturers who have learned to promote change every day, you will be prepared to create a true change event rather than just another project. You will create a context in which people feel that they are taking part in the creation of a new vision, not just tinkering with the old one.

Another requirement: agreed-on criteria for success (chapter 2). If they aren't careful, health care organizations can find themselves doing the wrong things right—doing a good job implementing something that should not or does not need to be done. They may wind up relying on inadequate measures, such as project scope, schedule, and budget, while ignoring critical elements, such as fitness for use. They may take on unnecessary risks or ignore necessary ones. Risk assessment is a key part of the first mile. It is one of the central elements that make for a smooth ride later on.

A third requirement: careful planning (chapter 3). No engineer would think of building a bridge without detailed studies and drawings showing exactly how it is to be constructed. A change event is essentially a bridge to the future—and it, too, needs detailed planning as to how it will work. One point to remember about planning is that it is cheap. It is easy to change a blueprint, a budget, or a plan of action before a project begins. Once the project is under way, however, change is far more difficult and usually much more expensive. Planning is also the best time for detailed analysis of potential failure. Health care organizations cannot afford real failure, because they run the risk of making people worse off. The planning stage is when you can answer the question, "If this initiative does not proceed as we expect, what is likely to happen?"

Note something important here. We have discussed three elements that are critical for the success of a change event—mind-set, success criteria, and planning—and nobody has yet begun to take action. We have selected no projects, chosen no people, created no project teams. These initial elements have to be baked into the organization's approach to change before it takes even the first step.

Then come the elements that enable the organization to actually launch a project.

One of these is deciding what it wants to do—in other words, creating and identifying the right initiatives (chapter 4). Most places do have plenty of ideas for change. But are they the right ones? Do they fit with the organization's mission, vision, and values (MV^2), and with its strategic plan? Successful organizations typically develop several techniques for identifying and encouraging ideas that do have the proper fit, such as listening sessions and gemba walks. They make it possible for people to develop their ideas, to turn them from seeds into sprouts. The *plan of concept* that results is not yet a detailed road map. But it answers the questions an organization needs to have answered before investing time and resources in exploring the idea.

Next comes the job of selecting, prioritizing, and monitoring change initiatives (chapter 5). Selection usually falls to a project and portfolio management review board (PPMRB), a select group of people from various parts of the organization whose job it is to launch and monitor change initiatives while also considering the entire pipeline. The PPMRB establishes criteria for projects and evaluates ideas according to those criteria. It prioritizes projects, so that the organization does not mindlessly embark on more initiatives than it can handle (as so many organizations do today). And it monitors projects throughout their life cycle, assessing their progress, approving additional phases when appropriate, and decommissioning projects when required. As I noted in chapter 5, an organization without a PPMRB is like an airport without a control tower. Little wonder that so many projects at these organizations never reach takeoff velocity.

Choosing the right people may be the single most important task associated with actually launching a project (chapter 6). And it can be very, very difficult. Everyone in a health care organization has plenty of demands on his or her time. In some cases only a few individuals may have the hard skills, such as clinical or financial expertise, required for particular projects. The so-called soft skills are usually more important than hard skills, and may be even rarer. Essential soft skills in a health care setting include the ability to hold crucial conversations, a high level of emotional intelligence, and the ability to trust and to inspire trust. If initiatives are to succeed, they must be staffed by people who have a high quotient of these skills.

Successful initiatives also need the right number and combination of people—not too many, not too few, and in the appropriate mix (chapter 7). For example, every group needs some right-brained people who can think creatively and some left-brained types who are good at hard-nosed analysis. The group needs both a project sponsor and a project implementation leader. It should have a skilled project assistant, who can keep things on track and free up other members of the group for substantive work. It needs a designated risk watcher, someone whose mission it is to watch for dark clouds on the horizon and to focus the group's attention on potential pitfalls. Successful organizations learn to create a "people inventory" showing the skills and experience each of their employees possesses, and they draw on this inventory when creating a project team.

Of course, the organization must then forge these people into a *real* team, not just a random collection of individuals (chapter 8). Project implementation leaders use such tools as onboarding and scripting the first meeting. They help the team determine how it will make decisions. The goal of such activities is not just to create a smoothly functioning working group; it is to put fire in people's bellies, to inspire the kind of passion and commitment that leads to real and sustained change. Change in a health care organization—perhaps in any organization—comes from creating emotional buy-in, not just from blueprints and analysis. It happens when people come to feel that they are on a journey with trusted colleagues toward a better future.

Health care needs results, not just effort. It needs change, not just plans and proposals. My hope is that this book will help you create effective change events. It is not the whole story by any means. But the first mile is the element on which everything else depends. Get started right, and the chances are good that you will finish right as well. I wish you the best of luck on your journeys.

SUMMARY

- Health care is changing rapidly, creating stress both for organizations and for the people who staff them. But organizations can take charge of that change by launching the right initiatives.

- The key to initiatives' success lies in the first mile: in adopting a new mind-set, in agreeing on criteria for success, and in careful planning.

- Then comes the job of deciding what the organization wants to do; selecting, prioritizing, and monitoring change initiatives; and building project teams with the right people. That is the path to great results.

INDEX